641.563 LU
Lund, JoAnna M.
H.E.L.P. : the healthy
exchanges lifetime plan : 6/97
SSP

South St. Paul Public Library
106 Third Avenue North
South St. Paul, MN 55075

H ◈ E ◈ L ◈ P™

Healthy Exchanges® Lifetime Plan

It's Not a Diet, It's a Way of Life®

Also by JoAnna M. Lund

Healthy Exchanges® Cookbook

The Diabetic's Healthy Exchanges® Cookbook

The Best of Healthy Exchanges® Food Newsletter '92 Cookbook

Notes of Encouragement

It's Not a Diet, It's a Way of Life®
(AUDIOTAPE)

H·E·L·P™

The Healthy Exchanges® Lifetime Plan

JoAnna M. Lund

with Barbara Alpert

G. P. PUTNAM'S SONS

New York

South St. Paul Public Library
106 Third Avenue North
South St. Paul, MN 55075

G. P. Putnam's Sons
Publishers Since 1838
200 Madison Avenue
New York, NY 10016

Copyright © 1996 by Healthy Exchanges, Inc.

Diabetic Exchanges Calculated by Rose Hoenig, R.D., L.D.

Before using the recipes and advice in this book, consult your physician or health care provider to be sure they are appropriate for you. The information in this book is not intended to take the place of any medical advice. It reflects the author's experiences, studies, research, and opinions regarding a healthy lifestyle. All material included in this publication is believed to be accurate. The publisher assumes no responsibility for any health, welfare, or subsequent damage that might be incurred from use of these materials.

No part of this book may be reproduced by any mechanical, photographic, or electronic process; or in the form of a phonographic recording; nor may it be stored in a retrieval system, transmitted, translated into another language, or otherwise copied for public or private use, excepting brief passages quoted for purposes of review, without the permission of the publisher and author.

For more information about Healthy Exchanges® products, contact:

Healthy Exchanges, Inc.
P.O. Box 124
DeWitt, Iowa 52742-0124
(319) 659-8234

Published simultaneously in Canada

Library of Congress Cataloging-in-Publication Data

Lund, JoAnna M.
HELP: the healthy exchanges lifetime plan : it's not a diet, it's a way of life / by JoAnna M. Lund, with Barbara Alpert.
p. cm.
Based on the author's bestselling original Healthy Exchanges cookbook.
ISBN 0-399-14164-2
1. Reducing diets—Recipes. 2. Food exchange lists. 3. Diabetes—Diet therapy—Recipes. 4. Coronary heart disease—Diet therapy—Recipes. I. Alpert, Barbara. II. Lund, JoAnna M. Healthy Exchanges cookbook. III. Healthy Exchanges, Inc. IV. Title.
RM222.2.L746 1997 95-25676 CIP
641.5'63—dc20

Book design by Richard Oriolo

Printed in the United States of America

5 7 9 10 8 6

This book is printed on acid-free paper. ♾

This book is dedicated in loving memory to my parents, Jerome and Agnes McAndrews. God has blessed me with my mother's creativity and writing talents and my father's analytical skills. He allowed their earthly abilities to bloom in me when I began my quest for a commonsense approach to lifelong healthy living.

I plan on riding my "Health Wagon" for life, and I want you to join me on this journey. The next time you think you can't get through another day without falling off the Health Wagon, read this poem my mother wrote several years before her death. It just may help you climb back on board for good.

Your Little Wagon

Did you ever try hitching
Your wagon to a star,
Then stopped because you thought
It a little too far?

Did the effort seem too hard
In achieving the gain
Your little wagon for you
Could someday obtain?

Did you think the star moved
Higher into the sky
When you let go of the reins
Without even a try?

Do not blame the star.
It did not move against your will.
It was you and your little wagon
That really stood still.

—AGNES CARRINGTON MCANDREWS

Acknowledgments

When you find something that works, that makes you feel better than you ever have in your life, you quickly jump on that bandwagon yourself—and then you share the good news with everyone you meet.

Because I plan on riding my "Health Wagon" for life, I want to make the journey as pleasant as possible. For riding along with me and keeping me going, I want to express my thanks:

To God, for giving me the talent to create Healthy Exchanges and the courage to keep trying through the trying times. With God's help, I've achieved more than I dreamed possible when I began.

To Cliff Lund, my truck-drivin' man. After more than four years of working together twenty-four hours a day in Healthy Exchanges endeavors, he still hasn't jumped off the Health Wagon. I could not do what I want to do without his unqualified support and encouragement.

To John Duff, my editor. He shared my vision and never tried to change me, my mainstream "common folk" healthy recipes and cooking techniques, or my "Grandma Moses" style of writing. He just helped me improve what I was doing naturally. You can't ask for more than that from anyone.

To Barbara Alpert, my writing associate. Within minutes of visiting with her, I realized that she could help me gather my thoughts, goals, and dreams on paper so that I could better share them with others. She captured me better than I could have alone. This truly is a case where two minds were better than one.

To Angela Miller and Coleen O'Shea, my agents. They took this small-town, middle-aged woman "as is" and never tried to change me into "big city." Their support and professionalism mean so much.

To Phyllis Grann, Susan Petersen, Donna Gould, Cathy Lee Gruhn, Barbara O'Shea, and the entire team at Putnam, who agreed that my commonsense approach to healthy living was a winning program that would appeal to a nationwide audience. They supplied some powerful ingredients in my recipe for success.

To Rose Hoenig, R.D., L.D., for computing the diabetic exchanges and answering my questions about healthy nutrition. Her help makes it possible for me to help so many others.

To Becky, James, Tommy, Pam, John, Zach, Josh, Mary, Regina, Marge, and Cleland. My children, grandchildren, sisters, and in-laws who have supported me and my efforts from the moment I scribbled that very first recipe down on my trusty legal pad. I don't know if I would have been brave enough to share what I was doing with others if they hadn't been so supportive.

To my Healthy Exchanges "family members" all over the world. Everyone who uses my recipes or lives by my commonsense approach to healthy living is part of my "family." If the family members hadn't shared their stories and successes with me, if they hadn't shown me that Healthy Exchanges could transform *their* lives as well as mine, this book would never have been written.

Traveling together makes the journey much more pleasant. Thank you for jumping on board, too. There is room enough for all of us.

Foreword

Helping you help yourself—that's the theme of HELP, the Healthy Exchanges Lifetime Plan. Have you been trying to live a healthier lifestyle? Are you interested in eating smart and controlling your fat and sugar intake? Healthy Exchanges recipes will help you accomplish these vital goals, as they have already done for thousands of readers of JoAnna Lund's cookbooks and newsletters.

If you want to pursue a healthier lifestyle, but you're not sure how to begin, HELP will provide a road map, showing you how incorporating healthy eating and moderate exercise into your daily routine can help you reach your goal of good health for a lifetime.

Use the information in this book, which is based on sound current nutrition practices and fitness guidelines, to design a plan that works for you. Take the time to monitor your progress, whether you're logging inches lost or blood glucose reports. Remember that no one plan works for everyone, so find the one that best suits your needs.

HELP can put you on the path to achieving a healthier lifestyle. Start making some positive changes today.

—Rose Hoenig, R.D., L.D.

Contents

Part Four

THE MENUS AND RECIPES

Introduction

How I Learned to HELP™ Myself:

JoAnna M. Lund and Healthy Exchanges®

For twenty-eight years I was the diet queen of DeWitt, Iowa. I tried every diet I ever heard of, every one I could afford, and every one that found its way to my small town in eastern Iowa. I was willing to try anything that promised to "melt off the pounds," determined to deprive my body in every possible way in order to become thin at last.

I sent away for expensive "miracle" diet pills. I starved myself on the liquid diets. I gobbled diet candies, took thyroid pills, fiber pills, prescription and over-the-counter diet pills. I went to endless weight-loss support-group meetings—but I managed to turn healthy programs such as Overeaters Anonymous, Weight Watchers, and TOPS into unhealthy diets . . . diets I could never follow for more than a few months.

I was determined to discover something that worked long-term, but each new failure increased my desperation that I'd never find it.

I ate strange concoctions and rubbed on even stranger potions. I agreed to be hypnotized. I tried reflexology and even had an acupuncture device stuck in my ear!

Does my story sound a lot like yours? I'm not surprised. No wonder the weight-loss business is a billion-dollar industry!

Every new thing I tried seemed to work—at least at first. And losing that first five or ten pounds would get me so excited, I'd believe that this new miracle diet would, finally, get my weight off for keeps.

Inevitably, though, the initial excitement wore off. The diet's routine and boredom set in, and I quit. I shoved the pills to the back of the medicine chest; pushed the cans of powdered shake mix to the rear of the kitchen cabinets; slid all the program materials out of sight under my bed; and once more I felt like a failure.

Like most dieters, I quickly gained back the weight I'd lost each time, along with a few extra "souvenir" pounds that seemed always to settle around my hips. I'd done the diet-lose-weight-gain-it-all-back "yo-yo" on the average of once a year. It's no exaggeration to say that over the years I've lost 1,000 pounds—and gained back 1,150 pounds.

Finally, at the age of forty-six I weighed more than I'd ever imagined possible. I'd stopped believing that any diet could work for me. I drowned my sorrows in sacks of cake donuts and wondered if I'd live long enough to watch my grandchildren grow up.

Something had to change.

I had to change.

Finally, I did.

I'm just over fifty now—and I'm 130 pounds less than my all-time high of close to 300 pounds. I've kept the weight off for more than four years. I'd like to lose another ten pounds, but I'm not obsessed about it. If it takes me two or three years to accomplish it, that's okay.

What I *do* care about is never saying hello again to any of those unwanted pounds I said good-bye to!

How did I jump off the roller coaster I was on? For one thing, I finally stopped looking to food to solve my emotional problems. But what really shook me up—and got me started on the path that changed my life—was Operation Desert Storm in early 1991. I sent three children off to the Persian Gulf war—my son-in-law, Matt, a medic in Special Forces; my daughter, Becky, a full-time college student and member of a medical unit in the Army Reserve; and my son James, a member of the Inactive Army Reserve reactivated as a chemicals expert.

Somehow, knowing that my children were putting their lives on the line got me thinking about my own mortality—and I knew in my heart the last thing they needed while they were overseas was to get a letter from home saying that their mother was ill because of a food-related problem.

The day I drove the third child to the airport to leave for Saudi Arabia, something happened to me that would change my life for the better—and forever. I stopped praying my constant prayer as a professional dieter, which was simply "Please, God, let me lose ten pounds by Friday." Instead, I began praying, "God, please help me not to be a burden to my kids and my family."

I quit praying for what I wanted and started praying for what I needed—and in the process my prayers were answered. I couldn't keep the kids safe—that was out of my hands—but I could try to get healthier to better handle the stress of it. It was the least I could do on the home front.

That quiet prayer was the beginning of the new JoAnna Lund. My initial goal was not to lose weight or create healthy recipes. I only wanted to become healthier for my kids, my husband, and myself.

Each of my children returned safely from the Persian Gulf war. But something didn't come back—the 130 extra pounds I'd been lugging around for far too long. I'd finally accepted the truth after all those agonizing years of suffering through on-again, off-again dieting.

There are no "magic" cures in life.

No "magic" potion, pill, or diet will make unwanted pounds disappear.

I found something better than magic, if you can believe it. When I turned my weight and health dilemma over to God for guidance, a new JoAnna Lund and Healthy Exchanges were born.

I discovered a new way to live my life—and uncovered an unexpected talent for creating easy "common folk" healthy recipes, and sharing my commonsense approach to healthy living. I learned that I could motivate others to change their lives and adopt a positive outlook. I began publishing cookbooks and a monthly food newsletter, and speaking to groups all over the country.

I like to say, "*When life handed me a lemon, not only did I make healthy, tasty lemonade, I wrote the recipe down!*"

What I finally found was not a quick fix or a short-term diet but a great way to live well for a lifetime.

I want to share it with you.

Part One

HELP AT LAST

Any woman who admits she's over fifty, once weighed three hundred pounds, and wolfed down four cake donuts in five minutes flat is going to tell you the truth about everything else!

One

Diets Don't Work, but HELP Does

Diets don't work. Everyone says so . . . yet whenever someone proposes a new one, many people follow it, hoping that they'll finally discover a way to lose weight and keep it off for good. I know—I've been on so many diets I can't remember them all.

I started my first diet when I was just eighteen and fresh out of high school. Even though my body weight was normal, I saw myself as fat and unattractive. I believed dieting was the only answer. At twenty-one, when I got married, I was almost thin.

By twenty-eight, I might have been described as pleasingly plump. I had three kids, along with the extra pounds to prove it! By thirty, I was anorexic, though we didn't call it that then. I existed on soda crackers, bananas, and water. Isn't that a scary thought? My shoulder blades stuck out as far as my breasts did! I starved myself to please my first husband, because I *felt* starved for love.

At thirty-three, I gained fifty pounds in three months while I was going through my divorce. I remember waking up one day and not having a single thing to wear that fit. Small-town Irish Catholic girls just didn't get divorced, and I felt like a failure—to my kids, my parents, and my husband. I "handled" all these painful feelings by numbing myself with food.

By the time I hit thirty-five, the year I married Cliff, I was almost thin again. I managed to keep my weight down until the bottom fell out of the farm market three years later. We had $1,300 monthly truck payments to make, and so Cliff went to long-haul trucking. He was gone anywhere from two to six weeks at a time. I devoted all my energies to work and my kids, and I kept eating so I wouldn't be lonely. Food became my comfort because Cliff wasn't around. I was thirty-eight, and I had become downright obese.

For the next few years, I would go up and down twenty to thirty pounds a year. I was a perpetual dieter, but I never really got anywhere. I was always going on and off diets, trying new ones as the seasons changed. The year my daughter, Becky, got married, I managed to lose seventy pounds, because I didn't want to embarrass her on her special day. But the minute the reception was over, I was back on food. Within six months I gained it all back—and then some.

Diets don't work. I learned this the hard way after almost thirty years of firsthand experience. On the last day of my last diet, I weighed a whopping 150 pounds more than I did on the first day of my first diet. I felt desperate (who wouldn't?) but it took a serious personal crisis for me to figure out how I could conquer my problem and get on with my life.

When I said good-bye to my son James at the airport that dreary January day in 1991, I tipped the scales at my all-time high of around three hundred pounds, sporting fifty-six-inch hips. I knew that in order to get through this extraordinarily difficult time, I could no longer cope by reaching for bags of cake donuts as I always had. Sitting alone in my car, I prayed to God for the strength to begin living a healthy lifestyle. My family had enough to worry about, especially now, and I didn't want to be an added burden. I decided it was time I stopped letting my health deteriorate because of my continued abuse of food.

I was a veteran of so many diets; I'd read it all and I knew it all. But this time something was different. *I* was different, and somehow my motivation had changed.

Think of it this way: You're going full speed ahead in one direction, and then immediately, in one second, your direction totally

I am one of the many people who are overweight and need to eat healthier. My husband feels that he must *have his desserts after every meal, and that has been my downfall. I want to do better, and so I have decided to invest in your books. Doctors say exercise and sometimes give food suggestions, but they don't teach you how to live day after day from morning until night.*

—M. B. E., WI

changes. As I was driving James down to the airport to leave for Saudi Arabia, I was not there yet. I was still a professional dieter. But coming back from the airport, I had undergone a change. I was no longer a dieter. I was just trying to find a workable solution to my problem. I had changed my goal from losing weight to recapturing my health.

That day, I really didn't care if I ever lost a pound. I didn't care anymore. What I cared about was getting my health back, so my kids, who were already in danger, would never get a call from the Red Cross telling them that their mother was in the hospital or dead because of my own self-abuse of my body.

I needed to find a workable solution based on everything I'd read, a solution that combined food and exercise. But at the same time I realized I had to set manageable, interim goals that I had a real chance of reaching. And I had to start treating myself with dignity and respect. No matter what size I was, I was a person of value, and by developing a positive attitude, I knew I would strengthen my self-esteem.

I *had* to do it.

I had to do it for my kids and Cliff.

No, I realized suddenly. I was doing it *for me*, but because of them.

I wasn't doing it to lose weight to look decent in a dress for Becky's wedding (I'd already done that). I wasn't dieting to get thinner so I wouldn't embarrass my son Tommy in front of his friends. I'd tried losing weight for other people, and it had only brought me heartache and frustration.

But I also wasn't willing to go without reasonable portions or never eat dessert again because James was worried I would get sick and die like his grandma. I wasn't going to swallow diet pills by the handful so Cliff wouldn't be embarrassed to be seen in public with me.

Normally, if people lose weight for other people, it's to gain their approval. This time, I wasn't doing it to please them, but it had everything to do with what they meant to me. Life was suddenly more precious, maybe, and the danger my children were facing overseas made me face up to the danger I faced myself.

GETTING STARTED ON THE ROAD TO HEALTH

I was a bundle of mixed emotions as I started living my healthy lifestyle. It was scary to put so much faith in myself, to believe I could do this. And yet it was uplifting at the same time, if that makes sense. I couldn't do a thing for the kids except pray, but I began to feel I had the power to get healthier and stronger, emotionally and physically, to better handle the stress in my life.

I knew I had to find a healthy way of eating, and a way to exercise. I was so heavy and so out of shape, there wasn't much I could do, other than walking (and this was January in Iowa, remember). That first day, when I came home from the airport, I parked the car and took a walk. As I walked, I began praying for answers, praying for the kids' safety. It literally took me about thirty-five to forty minutes to walk one mile, but I did it.

The next day I put my boots on and walked the eight blocks to work through the snow. It was a start. By the time I walked to work in the early morning and back at night, I'd put in almost a mile. Then I decided to walk to the grocery store, too. I would take my satchel and stop on my way home from work to pick up what I needed. On the weekends, I would *walk* to the store and do my shopping.

I also began walking in the early mornings up at our local health club, the Hart Center. I walked by myself, not listening to a radio but thinking and praying—for the kids to be safe, and for the strength to just do it right for one more day. (In the past, I'd gone to the club sporadically when I was in one of my diet modes, but this time was different. I was doing it for my health, instead of expecting an immediate result that showed on the scale.)

I would get up at five in the morning so I could be there at five-thirty, and I'd walk around and around the indoor track. Since I was walking so slowly, the only people who didn't pass me were the few using walkers or canes. Everyone else kept passing me, but I didn't care. I just kept going.

One lady, Millie, who is twenty-five years older than I am, and whose grandson is one of my son's best friends, always encouraged me as she whooshed by me on each lap. I vowed that someday I would walk as fast as she did. (It took me from January until

There are two good ways to get to the top of an oak tree: climb . . . or find a good acorn, sit on it, and wait.

April to walk at Millie's pace, but the day I could walk as fast as she did, the day I could finally keep up with her, I smiled from ear to ear all day long. When I think about it, it still puts a smile in my heart. I told her, after I could keep up with her, that she had been my only goal—and that made her smile from ear to ear too!)

The walking cleared my head, made my heart beat faster, and gave me time to think about how I could live my life in a healthier way. It also gave me a kind of satisfaction for another reason. I'd given the war effort three kids, and I was very clear about why we were over there: oil. I vowed I wasn't going to give any oil baron anywhere one extra cent. They had my kids; they weren't getting my money. Sometimes decisions we make on principle inspire us to do things we wouldn't do otherwise. In this case, it was an extra, added push to leave the car home.

People don't think diet and dessert are in the same "D" section of the dictionary, but they are if they're Healthy Exchanges recipes. They're not with "dreadful" or "dull" but with "delightful" and "delicious."

Eating for My Health

I started fixing my own foods, making up healthy and satisfying versions of dishes I enjoyed. In my old dieting days, I would have gotten along on whatever tiny amount of food someone else told me to eat. Now I knew I needed the fuel and energy, for work, for school, for my kids, and for the exercise I was doing.

I would cook for the whole week on Sunday because I knew I wouldn't have time during the week. I worked forty hours a week, and I was taking twelve hours of credits at college that semester. When I wasn't at work or at school, I was glued to CNN to find out what was happening to my kids. So I didn't have time for cooking, and I *knew* I wasn't going to have time anytime soon.

From the very first day, I was sure of two things. First, if I was going to get Cliff's cooperation, I had to figure out what kinds of food I could prepare *that he would eat* along with me. If it was Mexican, Italian, meat and potatoes, or dessert, I knew he would be more likely than not to give it a chance.

The second thing I knew was that dessert was important to me. My mother had always served dessert. She was an outstanding cake baker and made the most wonderful pies and cookies, so that desserts were a real part of what made me feel cozy, connected, and close with my mother. She had died just months before I sent my first soldier off to war, and she was my last parent. I felt that I needed the comfort and coziness that eating dessert was going to give me. So from the very beginning I decided to prepare and enjoy a healthy dessert *every day of my life.*

Look, when I'm really hungry, carrot sticks and vegetable salad are not going to do the trick. They might keep me from whatever else I wanted for about ten minutes, but after that I'd be right back reaching for sweets, because even though I'd fed my stomach, I hadn't fed my soul.

Instead, if I ate a piece of dessert, or had a tasty snack, I wouldn't gobble down an overabundance of other things. Instead of using large quantities of salad and vegetables to stuff myself, I even learned to eat vegetables in moderation.

GOING "PUBLIC"

As part of my new healthy eating plan, I began taking my lunch to work. When I laid it out in front of me, the ladies I was eating with thought what I had looked better than what they had purchased or brought from home, and they started picking off my plate. (Let me say that about the only bad habit I never acquired was taking food off other people's plates. If someone else drank out of a glass or took a bite off my plate, however, I was done with it. I couldn't touch it if I was starving. That meant that I couldn't eat the rest of what I'd brought with me.)

So the next day I brought two lunches, one for me and one for them. Any day I figured I had something they'd want to try, I just packed an extra serving for them to taste. Every time I brought one of my new "creations," my co-workers asked for the recipe.

That's really how Healthy Exchanges got started, just that informally. The proof was clearly in the tasting of the pudding (or the salad or the pie), and it seemed that almost every day someone was copying one of my recipes down.

I'd worked with some of these people for eighteen years. They'd seen my weight go up and down and up and down, again and again. They knew the stress I was under now, and that I usually handled stress by eating.

But this was the first time they saw me consistently keep losing

The truth is, I've dieted myself fat. Now I'm interested in learning how to cook foods I can eat, enjoy, and not blimp out on. Today I'm ready to get on with my life and learn how to be good to me.

—R. B., IL

pounds, without ever feeling deprived. I was eating the best food in the place, and the most food, too.

(By *most,* I don't mean an overabundance, just realistic portions of real foods. I wasn't eating a handful of carrot sticks with diet soda as a chaser and calling it a meal anymore. But I also wasn't going to eat a whole casserole and call it a snack. Then, as now, I understood that *moderation* was the key.)

Learning proper portion control was probably one of the hardest things for me to do. But because I was eating good food in reasonable amounts now, I found that I could eat what I needed and not go overboard.

Just Doing It

That's how I began. I walked every day, and I kept creating recipes that satisfied my tummy and my soul as well. I would take about three or four hours every Sunday doing my cooking marathon, so I could open the door of the freezer each night after work, and good-tasting food that was *good* for me would be waiting there.

It worked. It was the most stressful time of my life, but because I had decided to start living healthily, I felt less stressed and more hopeful than I had in years.

I wasn't willing to make short-term sacrifices anymore in hopes of losing a few pounds. I was looking at living this way long-term . . . beyond however long the war lasted, not just until the kids came home. I knew immediately I was going to be doing this the rest of my life.

The eating plan I called Healthy Exchanges and the four-part HELP program that followed grew out of weeks and months of figuring out what worked for me. I didn't share it with anyone for a while. I had decided to attend a weight-loss group for the initial support, and was basically following their program, but from the very first day I began creating my own recipes. Even though I was coping with all my stress and difficult times, everyone wanted to sit next to me. I kept filling the people next to me with the motivation to keep going, sharing my philosophy with them—"Don't think of this as a diet, don't worry about what the scale says, do this because you're feeling good, do it because it's the healthy thing to do." I would get the people around me so pumped up, they would all be back the next week. It was literally like musical chairs to see who was going to sit next to me!

Before long, people in town were stopping me to say that they needed a "fix" of whatever I was doing, and I would freely share my ideas with them. That's how I started defining the Healthy Exchanges Lifetime Plan. I discovered I'd been living it from the very first day without realizing what I was doing.

You're the best thing that has come into my life since my granddaughter was born, and I mean that with all my heart! I've lost eighty-five pounds and am still continuing to lose. I'm so happy I have someone to share the same problem with. I've battled overweight for more years than I care to admit. Now I know I'm going to reach my goal—and I have you and the Lord to thank for it.

—C. H., OH

Reaching for Better Health

I soon found that my new way of living delivered other rewards besides weight loss and renewed energy. Within a month of changing my lifestyle, I no longer had to take gout medicine. I had been spending sixty dollars a month to keep my big toe from throbbing as it hit my shoe. I wanted to be able to throw that gout medicine away. And I wanted to be able to get my blood tested and have my triglycerides within the normal range. After only a month, I managed to do both.

That really felt wonderful. I was finally living in a healthy way, not in a dieting way. And I'd done it for myself.

My doctor had been preaching to me for years about my excess weight. Every time I went for a checkup, I was usually a different weight. Then, about a month before I sent my kids off to war, the doctor told me if I didn't do something pretty fast, I was on the brink of really jeopardizing my health. She told me to come back at the end of January to be retested, and when I did—after living healthily for just a month—I no longer needed the gout medicine and my triglycerides were in the normal range.

The nurse gave me a copy of the test and I brought it home as a souvenir—and a badge of honor. I could use the money I saved from not having to buy the gout medicine to pay the phone bills when the kids had a chance to call collect from overseas. It was important to me to keep the family connected.

Ask, and it shall be given you; Seek, and ye shall find; Knock, and it shall be opened unto you: For every one that asketh receiveth; And he that seeketh findeth; And to him that knocketh it shall be opened.

—Jesus of Nazareth

Asking for Help

But that doesn't mean every single day was easy. Some days were a lot easier than others, while still others were a real struggle. No single day, though, was 100 percent difficult, because every day I said the same prayer that I still say now. My daily prayer was and is "Dear God, help me help myself just for today."

I really do say that prayer every day. But I firmly believe that prayers alone are not going to do it. You can pray for a miracle, but you have to do your part too. I also believe that the effort alone won't do it long-term. Prayers, coupled with your best effort, are almost certain to produce a good final result.

My husband, Cliff, was an important reason I was able to make my new lifestyle work. I'd started out to find a solution for me that would be workable for him, and because he saw me reaching out to him for his cooperation, he gave it fully. In fact, he told me that as long as I kept creating recipes that tasted as good as mine did, he'd eat anything I put in front of him—well, with the exception of anything with broccoli in it!

The weight-loss support group I attended for a while also helped. I'd hoped that being around others who had the same concerns would help me through those difficult first weeks. I joined the class the same week I put my third soldier on the plane for Saudi Arabia. It was January and the room was packed. I remember when the leader asked if anyone was under any extra stress, and I started crying. I said yes, that even as we were talking my kids could be in danger. The very next day I got a letter in the mail from the leader, telling me that her heart went out to me, and that anytime I needed any extra help or support, not to hesitate to call her at home. I've never forgotten her. (She gets a complimentary copy of my newsletter for the rest of her life.)

I think that's one of the reasons I try so hard, that I do my best to reach out to people who need help now. Because she was there when I needed her, Cliff was there when I needed him, and God definitely lightened the load when I needed it. So now I want to give back hope to people who need it most.

Help yourself, and heaven will help you.

—La Fontaine

Helping You to Help Yourself

What began as my personal journey in search of a healthier lifestyle evolved into the Healthy Exchanges Lifetime Plan—or HELP, for short—a combination of Healthy food, moderate Exercise, Lifetime changes, and a Positive attitude. If any part of the H-E-L-P is missing, it's still just a diet. By choosing to follow the HELP way of life, you'll be able to lose weight and keep it off, lower cholesterol, and control or lessen the effects of diabetes.

How does the Healthy Exchanges Lifetime Plan work?

H—Healthy eating is the first step. I'll give you recipes for delicious "real-people" food that is low in fat and sugar, dishes your entire family can enjoy together. No longer will you have to prepare one meal for the "dieter" and another for the rest of the family. The Healthy Exchanges Lifetime Plan provides all you need to plan and prepare healthy meals every day, from helping you plan menus and shop for the ingredients in your local market to offering healthy tips on eating out and entertaining. At the heart of the HELP eating plan are my recipes—dozens of them—from soups and salads to main dishes and irresistible desserts. You won't have to sacrifice flavor anymore in order to lose weight—which is the key to sticking with this healthy eating program.

E—Regular, moderate **Exercise** that you enjoy will soon become a part of your daily routine. I alternate between walking, bicycling, and water aerobics, but your personal choice is up to you. I'll present an easy-to-follow plan to help you identify the exercises that fit your lifestyle and then offer some helpful ways to develop and monitor your daily exercise goals.

L—Setting **Lifetime** goals and being willing to make real changes in the way you live your life are the keys to making your success a lasting one. HELP is not a "diet" you start and finish. It is a way of life for you and your family, one you can be comfortable

JoAnna, you have been such a God-given wonder that words in a letter don't seem to be enough. You're an inspiration wherever you go.

—S. F., IA

with and enjoy for the rest of your lives. I'll show you how to make changes that will put more "Life" in your lifestyle and more years of good health in your lifetime.

P—Positive attitude is the final piece of the plan. It means accepting yourself for the wonderful, unique person you are, and that God meant you to be. For me, this is the key to living the HELP lifestyle to the fullest. Life doesn't begin when a woman squeezes into a size 10, or when a man fits into jeans with a 32-inch waist. If you need to lose weight, lower your cholesterol, or stabilize your blood sugar, you know it won't happen instantly. But by taking life one day at a time, by doing the best you can, by living your life as fully as possible—you can begin right now to make Positive changes in your life. The Healthy Exchanges Lifetime Plan will show you how to develop and practice the habit of positive thinking, including a special Positive Action Diary to help you begin.

Remember, if any part of H-E-L-P is missing, it's just another diet!

Since I began speaking to groups about HELP just over three years ago, tens of thousands have responded to its commonsense lifestyle advice. Not only have they used the plan to lose weight, lower cholesterol, and control blood sugar, they've developed stronger self-esteem and feel great about themselves!

But Isn't HELP a Diet?

I consider "diet" to be a four-letter word. It's downright obscene. Do you remember the cartoon that told us that the first three letters of diet are D-I-E? I know it's how I felt sometimes when forced to contemplate the "diet" dish before me! We weren't meant to live on liquid meals, or special powders, or beans at every meal. Diets are based on deprivation. They require us to alter our lives, dictate small amounts of strange foods, and deaden our taste buds to the pleasure of eating.

Typical diet plans make it necessary to prepare two separate meals: the first, a skimpy, go-without meal for the dieter (the family will usually turn up their noses at it) and another that features traditional favorites, "real-people" food for the rest of the family. If you've been a perennial dieter, you've probably had to do this more than once—and I'm sure you remember the moment when you'd had enough of the diet you were struggling to follow. You were preparing the family's "real-people" meal, and you sampled it just to make sure it was okay. That one sample led to another, and then another. Ultimately, you said the heck with it, guiltily ate dinner with the family, and vowed that you'd start the diet again tomorrow.

But of course tomorrow never comes, and you acknowledge another diet defeat. I had a string of such defeats, and each one left me feeling more angry and helpless. And so many of the dieters I've spoken with share such feelings about their dieting failures.

Now, be honest. How many of these "tricks" have you pulled in the past that indicate you're *just dieting?*

- Have you attended a weight-loss group and gone without food the day of your weigh-in, then devoured everything in sight as soon as the meeting was over?
- Have you gotten on the scale two or three times a day to check your weight (I know some who've weighed themselves on the hour!) instead of only once a week?
- Have you fallen off your diet because you've been preparing foods for your family that were too tempting to resist?
- Have you been waiting until after you lose weight to live your life fully and do the things you really enjoy? Have you put off making each day an adventure?

If you answered "yes" to any of these questions, then you are still *just dieting!* If you are still just dieting, I suspect you'll probably never lose the weight you want to, and keep it off for good. Not until you throw the dieting "monkey" off your back.

I began by sharing my message through my newsletter, and many people said it was like getting a letter from a good friend once a month, a friend who *talks from the heart*. I've written this book so you won't have to wait for my letters but can keep me on your kitchen shelf or even on the night table for when you feel like having a friend to share your journey to better health.

In the old days, if I didn't lose ten pounds in two weeks, I'd consider the diet a failure, go off it, and gain back everything I'd lost—plus a few extra pounds for good measure. But when I finally quit

Whatever the hand findeth to do, do it with all thy might.

—Old Testament

"just dieting," my body began to do what it had failed to do when I was a professional dieter. Yes, it may take two months instead of two weeks to lose ten pounds, but the chances are much better that when those ten pounds come off, they won't come back. Changing *my* expectations about weight loss helped me finally end my battle with all those diets—and win the weight-loss war.

Now it's your turn!

Accept the current reality.
Create your vision.
Take action.
—P. E., OH

Two

From Healthy Exchanges to HELP

Every success story begins somewhere, and maybe the story of Healthy Exchanges really began more than a decade ago when I was still a "professional dieter." A colleague at work passed along a recipe for a diet casserole, one that she told me "really isn't too bad." On one of those rare nights when everyone was home for dinner—the kids weren't off at some school activity, and Cliff was not on the road—I decided to try it.

The kids took one bite and said in unison, "Yuck, Mom, what's this junk?" Then Cliff tasted it, pushed his plate away, and stood up. "Come on, kids," he said, "if your mom wants to eat this [and I'm cleaning up his language here] diet 'slop,' that's okay. But we don't have to!" They headed off to the nearest pizza parlor, leaving me all alone to face my unappetizing, tasteless diet "slop."

After that, I had to prepare two separate meals when I was on a diet—real food for them, and *diet slop* for me. I ate that tasteless casserole all by myself because I was gung-ho on a diet at the time. But days later I was downing a whole pizza (not to mention a

Don't be afraid of a new idea. Even a turtle knows he must stick his neck out to get anywhere.

—S. Q., OH

sack of cake donuts for dessert) because I couldn't stick with that diet slop for more than a few days. So what did that diet slop really cost me? First, I threw most of it away because my family wouldn't eat it and I couldn't stand it for more than a couple of days. Second, I lost the precious time of sharing a meal with my family because they chose to eat elsewhere rather than suffer through that casserole with me. Third, any temporary weight loss that occurred because of my eating that diet dish was quickly replaced by a weight gain when I went back to my old eating habits in less than a week. And perhaps most important, my self-esteem took another nosedive when I couldn't stick with the diet. The tangible and intangible expenses of that particular meal will forever be part of my memories.

But I owe that woman a vote of thanks because her "not-too-bad" casserole propelled me into action, even if it took another ten years before I understood why I couldn't live that way anymore—preparing one meal for my family and another for me. I had to figure out how to feed all of us at once, but I couldn't spend hours creating magic in the kitchen. I needed food that could be prepared quickly, when I got home after work—I didn't have endless time to weigh and measure and make separate meals, as many diets force you to.

I began to look for healthy recipes and to plan menus that the entire family would eat with enthusiasm. Out of that search came Healthy Exchanges, a way of eating that changed all our lives.

What Healthy Exchanges Means

Is it really possible to enjoy favorite foods once the excess sugars and fats are removed? Yes, and I can prove it to you—just as I proved to myself and my family that I could create healthy recipes that tasted like "real food."

When I came up with the concept for Healthy Exchanges, I had three ideas in mind:

1. I wanted to "**exchange**" old, unhealthy habits for new, healthy ones in food, exercise, and mental attitude.

2. I chose to "**exchange**" ingredients within each recipe to eliminate as much fat and sugar as possible, while retaining the original flavor, appearance, and aroma.

3. I calculated all recipes using the **exchange** system of measuring daily food intake as established by the American Dietetic Association, the American Diabetic Association, and many national weight-loss organizations.

There's a real-life example of how it works on page 18: I took my mother's favorite no-bake cheesecake recipe (delicious but *very* high in fat and sugar!) and created a Healthy Exchanges version that will persuade just about anyone that they're eating a luscious, rich dessert. (You'll also notice how much easier the preparation is for my "creation.")

I wanted to let you know what a lifesaver your book has been for me. The recipes are so easy, and the desserts are incredible. When I tell people what I eat—the pies, the dessert salads—they look incredulous, but I've lost more than sixty pounds since February. And I've never felt so satisfied in my life!

—M. F., MI

Mother's No-Bake Cheesecake

2 envelopes unflavored gelatin
1 cup sugar
¼ teaspoon salt
2 eggs, separated
1 cup milk
1 teaspoon grated lemon peel
3 cups creamed cottage cheese
1 teaspoon lemon juice
1 tablespoon vanilla extract
1½ cups graham cracker crumbs
¼ cup brown sugar
6 tablespoons melted butter
1 cup heavy cream or whipping cream
Strawberries, sliced peaches, chopped nuts, or canned fruit for garnish

Early in the Day or Before Serving: In a medium saucepan, stir gelatin with salt and sugar. In a small bowl, beat egg yolks with milk until mixed; stir into gelatin mixture. Cook over medium heat, stirring occasionally, until mixture thickens and coats the spoon. Remove from heat; add lemon peel; cool.

Press cottage cheese through a sieve into a large bowl. Stir in lemon juice, vanilla, and gelatin mixture. Refrigerate 30 minutes, stirring frequently, or until mixture mounds slightly when dropped from the spoon.

Meanwhile, combine graham cracker crumbs, brown sugar, and butter. Press half of it in the bottom of a 9-inch springform pan.

In a small bowl, with mixer at high speed, whip egg whites just until stiff peaks form. In a small bowl, whip cream until soft peaks form. With a rubber spatula, fold egg whites and whipped cream into the gelatin mixture; pour into pan. Sprinkle top with remaining crumb mixture and chill until firm.

To Serve: Remove side of pan. With large spatula, loosen cake from pan bottom; slide onto plate. Garnish with your choice of fruit or nuts.

Cut into 10 servings.

There are 543 calories and 27 grams of fat for just a small piece of Mom's cheesecake! It tasted good, but not good enough to use up that many fat grams.

Healthy Exchanges Lemon Lane Cheesecake with Blueberry Glaze

Here's my makeover of this tasty dish, with most of the fat and sugar gone—but the delicious flavor remains!

2 (8-ounce) packages Philadelphia fat-free cream cheese
1 (4-serving) package Jell-O sugar-free instant vanilla pudding mix
1 (4-serving) package Jell-O sugar-free lemon gelatin
⅔ cup Carnation nonfat dry milk powder
1 cup Diet Mountain Dew soda
*¾ cup Cool Whip Lite**
1 (6-ounce) Keebler butter-flavored piecrust
½ cup blueberry spreadable fruit

To Prepare: In a large bowl, stir cream cheese with a spoon until soft. Add dry pudding mix, dry gelatin, dry milk powder, and Diet Mountain Dew. Mix well using a wire whisk. Blend in ¼ cup Cool Whip Lite. Spread mixture evenly in piecrust. Chill 10 minutes. Place blueberry spreadable fruit in a 1-cup glass measuring cup and microwave on High for 30 seconds. Mix well. Evenly spread warm spreadable fruit on top of cheesecake. Refrigerate at least two hours. When ready to serve, top each piece with 1 tablespoon Cool Whip Lite.

Makes 8 servings.

The Healthy Exchanges version sounds delicious enough, doesn't it? But here's some information that will make it taste even better. The traditional version has 27 grams of fat per slice, and 543 calories per serving. The Healthy Exchanges piece (which is larger!) has just 6 grams of fat and 251 calories per slice.

Have I whetted your appetite? Just wait—I've only begun to show you how common sense and a passion for good eating led me to create Healthy Exchanges. But this book will give you much more than a collection of healthy, good-for-you, good-to-eat recipes.

* The ingredient is divided.

HELP is a plan that can help you accomplish your healthy living goals, whatever they are. Maybe you want to eat healthily. Or maybe you need to lose a few pounds—or a few more than that. But you need to find delicious, easy-to-make recipes the rest of the family will eat without objection. The dieter or health-conscious person may be willing to accept uninspired, low-fat, low-sugar "diet" recipes—but what can you do when your kids want pizza and your husband insists on hot-fudge sundaes and pie?

Most diet recipes deserve their bad reputations. Too many of them sacrifice taste and appeal for lower calories and less sodium or sweetener. That's usually why nobody likes to eat them—and why even if we stick to this kind of eating for a while, we eventually jump off the wagon!

This book will change all that—and change it for good. Ever since I began creating recipes, I have aimed for what I call "common folk healthy"—meaning that the recipes I create have to fit into an already-busy lifestyle, they have to consider our likes and dislikes as a family, and they have to appeal to everyone sitting at my table.

I do not shop at health-food stores, and I don't like preparing complicated dishes that keep me in the kitchen for hours. I got tired of being left with a pile of dirty dishes to show for all my efforts once the family had bolted from the table after a mere ten minutes. People may laugh when I say, *"If it takes longer to fix it than it does to eat it, forget it"*—but you'll be amazed to discover that you can eat well *and* healthily without spending hours cooking, chopping, and cleaning up!

My goal is this: The foods that I prepare have to look, taste, smell, and feel like the foods we have always enjoyed. Because I figured out how to "exchange" the excess fats and sugars within each recipe with readily available healthy ingredients, you'll be able to enjoy "real-food" dishes like lasagna, mashed potatoes, and strawberry cheesecake. (See Part Four: The Menus and Recipes for details!) Besides reducing the overall fat and sugar content, I lowered the sodium, too.

Using my recipes can help you lose weight, lower and control your cholesterol and/or blood sugar levels, and still allow you to enjoy delicious foods that deliver good nutrition and great "eye" appeal!

I didn't set out to impress anyone with fancy gourmet recipes that require unusual ingredients. Most of the mail I receive from

I have tons of recipes from a national weight loss organization but they call for ingredients I usually don't have in the house—or never use again.

—R. G., OR

people who've tried my recipes tells me that I made the right decision. They wanted (as my family and I did) to discover quick, tummy-pleasing, "common folk" dishes that are healthy, too—and in my Healthy Exchanges recipes they found exactly what they were looking for.

My sister Jeanie is another good example of the Healthy Exchanges recipe user. She could probably best be described as a "noncooking" cook. If a recipe isn't easy, she doesn't want to be bothered, because she has more important things to do with her time. But she gladly takes the few minutes required to stir up her favorite Healthy Exchanges recipes!

First say to yourself what you would be, and then do what you have to do.

—Epictetus

The Four "Musts"

Before I included any recipe in this book, it had to meet my Four "Musts." I knew that if I didn't address these "Musts" from the very beginning, I would be *just dieting* and only days or minutes away from falling off the Health Wagon, as I call it—and into a binge where I would be keeping company again with cake donuts and hot-fudge sundaes (my personal favorites . . . and downfalls!).

By eliminating unnecessary preparation and excess "bad" foods, I've made it much easier to live and eat healthily. Each of my recipes must be:

1. **Healthy**. Every recipe is low in fat and sugar and within a reasonable range for sodium. And because it is all these, it is also low in calories and cholesterol. The prepared food can be eaten with confidence by diabetics and heart patients as well as anyone interested in losing weight or maintaining a weight loss.

2. **Easy to make.** Most people don't have the time or the inclination to deal with complicated recipes. They just want to prepare something quickly and get it on the table as fast as possible. But they still want their families to be smiling when they leave the table. Simply put, they want dishes that are quick and easy to prepare—but that don't look as though they are!

3. **As tasty and good as it looks.** If the foods we eat don't look, taste, smell, and feel like the family favorites we are used to eating, we won't be willing to eat them week in and week out.

   We are all creatures of habit. If we grew up eating fried chicken with mashed potatoes every Sunday at noon, we may try poached chicken with plain potatoes once—but we'll go running back to our favorite greasy chicken as soon as we can. However, if we could enjoy healthy yet delicious oven-fried chicken with healthy yet satisfying mashed potatoes topped with rich, thick, healthy gravy, we would probably agree to give up the deep-fried chicken dinner. Rather than demanding that we give up a beloved comfort food but instead serving a healthy version with all the great flavor of the original dish we remember, we can feel satisfied—and willing to make this "Healthy Exchange" for the rest of our lives.

   Here's another example: "Good enough" will never be good enough for me again. My food has to be garnished in easy yet attractive ways so I feed my eyes as well as my stomach. That's why I sprinkle two tablespoons of chopped pecans on top of my **Almost Sinless Sundae Pie** (see page 268). The pie serves eight, which works out to about ⅔ teaspoon of nuts per person. But we definitely taste that crunch as we enjoy that piece of pie. And those delectable bites of pecan help keep us from gobbling handfuls of nuts while watching TV. It's when we think we can't have something that we *dwell* on it constantly until we do get it. Moderation is the cornerstone of Healthy Exchanges recipes. My recipes include tiny amounts of mini chocolate chips, coconut, miniature marshmallows, nuts, and other foods I like to call "real-people" foods—not so-called "diet" food. This is just one of the distinctions that set my cookbook apart from others emphasizing low-fat and/or low-sugar foods.

4. **Made from ingredients found in DeWitt, Iowa.** If the ingredients can be found in a small town with a population of 4,500 in the middle of an Iowa cornfield, then anyone ought to be able to find them, no matter where he or she shops! To make these recipes, you do not have to drive to a specialty

Feed your eyes, not your thighs.

store in a large city or visit a health-food store in search of special ingredients.

The servings that the recipes call for are ample for my husband and me, with enough left over for another meal or my husband's lunch the next day. Your recipes have made it much easier for us to eat well and practice weight control. The cost per recipe is very economical.

—B.W., IA

Making It Quickly, Easily, and More . . .

Once a recipe passes the Four Musts, I have a few additional requirements. One includes using the entire can if the container has to be opened with a can opener. The reason for this is simple: only a few people are perfect Suzy and Homer Homemakers; most of you are like me. If a recipe called for ⅓ cup tomato sauce, I would put the rest in the refrigerator with good intentions of using it up within a day or two—and six weeks later would probably have to toss it out because it was covered with moldy globs of green stuff. When I create a recipe, I devise a way to use the entire can and still have the dish taste delicious (and add up right when it comes to the mathematics of the exchanges for each serving).

Another test is what I call **"Will It Play in Anytown, USA?"** I ask myself if the retired person living on a meager pension or the young bride living on a modest paycheck can afford to prepare the recipe in terms of both equipment and ingredients. I ask myself if the person with arthritic hands or the mother with two small children underfoot can physically manage to make the recipe. If the answers are yes, that recipe will be included in my cookbooks or newsletters.

It's important to me that my recipes be simple to make and understand.

Here are some of the ways I do this:

- Wherever practical, I provide both the weight and the closest cup or spoon measurement for each ingredient. Why? Well, everyone who follows the major diet plans or uses the American Diabetic Association program is required to use a kitchen scale every day. But I know that in the real world this just doesn't happen. People say they're too busy to pull the scale out of the cupboard. Or they'd rather not use the measuring bowl and have to wash it. So my recipe says that 3 ounces of shredded reduced-fat cheese is equivalent to ¾ cup. I've measured this so often to make sure it's right. Why should you have to as well?

- I measure the final product and give the closest cup measurement per serving for anything that can't be cut into exact portions. For example, in a soup recipe, the serving size might be 1½ cups.
- I suggest baking all casseroles in an 8-by-8-inch pan for ease of portion control. If the dish serves 4, just cut it down the center, turn the dish, and cut it down the center again. Each cut square yields one serving. Many cookbooks call for a 1½-quart casserole, but I find that most people tend to scoop out too much or too little while the rest of the casserole collapses into the center. There's no guesswork my way—just an easy and accurate way to manage portion size.

To change my life, I must first change my thinking.

MEASURING SUCCESS ONE EXCHANGE AT A TIME

Healthy Exchanges recipes are unique for another reason: they provide nutritional information calculated in three ways:

1. ***Weight Loss Choices***®/*Exchanges.* The recipes can be used by anyone attending the national weight-loss programs or support groups that count daily food intake by exchanges or selections instead of calories.
2. ***Calories, Fat Grams, and Fiber.*** I list the fat grams right next to the calories. In traditional recipes, fat grams usually appear in the middle of the nutrient information. Now, if a person chooses to count fat grams or compare the percentage of fat calories to total calories, the information is quickly found. I also include fiber grams so you can monitor your fiber intake if you choose to.

I had to write and send a big hug and a thank-you! I've tried and tried everything. I'm surprised my husband agreed to do this with me. He has seen me up and down and he likes me up better. But these recipes and the healthy way they're made convinced him. I made a week's worth of menus. I've never spent so little for the three of us! I am finally happy. Your meals are excellent and I feel fantastic! No more yecky feeling from a lot of fat!

—D. M., MI

3. ***Diabetic Exchanges.*** A registered dietitian has calculated the Diabetic Exchanges to conform to the guidelines established by the American Diabetic Association. This makes this book a wonderful resource for diabetics, for those who need to cook for diabetic family members, and for professionals who educate diabetics in how to eat healthfully and control their condition.

I've provided these three different kinds of nutritional measurements to make it easier for anyone and everyone to use my recipes as part of their commitment to a healthy lifestyle. I will do just about anything to make cooking healthier and easier for people—except do their dishes!

Is Healthy Exchanges for You?

Do you want to lose weight— and keep it off for good?

I am living proof that you can lose weight while eating dishes prepared from Healthy Exchanges recipes. I went from a much-too-tight size 28 to a healthy size 12 to 14 by eating my own creations. I always make sure the bases are covered when it comes to meeting nutritional needs, and *then* I throw in tiny amounts of delicious treats—foods like mini chocolate chips that are usually considered "no-no's" in traditional diet recipes. Yes, we can get by without these little touches, but do we want to? Should we have to?

When I was a "professional" dieter, a typical lunch would consist of a couple of slices of diet bread, tuna packed in water, diet mayonnaise, lettuce, a glass of skim milk, and a small apple. Good healthy choices, all of them. But why was I always reaching for a candy bar or cake donuts just an hour later? Because I had fed only my stomach, and not my heart, my eyes, or my soul. It was only when I began enjoying a healthy piece of a real dessert every day that I began to lose weight and keep it off permanently. When I finally said NO to diets, I said YES to lasting weight loss!

The cardinal sin most people commit when going on a diet is preparing two different meals—skimpy, get-the-weight-off-as-fast-as-possible food for the dieter and real food for the rest of the family. My recipes can be eaten with confidence by anyone who wants to lose weight, but they are so tasty the entire family will gladly eat the same food. (I call it passing the "Cliff Lund Taste Test!") When you cook with Healthy Exchanges, the burden of preparing two separate meals, not to mention the temptation of "sampling" the good stuff to be sure "it tastes right," has been eliminated. Now instead of short-term dieting and weight loss that never seems to last, you can take a step forward to healthy living for a lifetime!

My husband is not only diabetic, he had a bypass surgery last December, so you can see that we have to change a lot of old habits to improve our health and keep it that way. I really like the recipes using foods that we used to use before we started falling apart as we reached our sixties. Thanks for the help I've been wanting and not finding in other cookbooks!

—M. R., IA

Are you a heart disease patient? Or do you just need to lower or limit cholesterol?

My Healthy Exchanges recipes are all low in fat, just right for you if you're recovering from a heart attack or if improving your cholesterol count is your goal. I have a recipe for Easy Lasagna Casserole which calls for real ingredients (*not* dietetic) and contains only 327 calories with 8 grams of fat per serving. It tastes just as good as a traditional recipe which delivers three times the amount of fat and almost twice the calories. And I don't skimp on the serving size! My approach provides a real savings in calories and fat without sacrificing flavor. While my own blood pressure and cholesterol are both within normal range, I know how important it is to stick to a diet low in fat. My parents both died of heart complications, so I'm particularly concerned about fat intake. This program provides dozens of delicious low-fat recipes to help you reach the best health possible.

In one month my husband lost nine pounds, and I lost four. His blood-sugar level went down 123 points due to your recipes.

—S. M., IL

Are you diabetic? Do you have hypoglycemia?

My recipes are also low in sugar. A typical serving of coconut-banana chocolate cream pie prepared in the traditional way provides approximately 504 calories with 26 grams of fat per serving, because processed sugar is the primary ingredient and fat not too far behind. My recipe for this pie (**Dwayne's Coconut Banana**

Chocolate Cream Pie, page 271) is *207 calories per serving* with only 7 grams of fat—and just because I banished excess fats and sugars doesn't mean I've sacrificed any flavor. Besides, my pie can be cut into 8 pieces instead of the usual 12 servings per pie suggested in many diet recipes. (Did you know that one-sixth of a pie used to be the standard-size serving? Now, too many recipes expect you to settle for one-twelfth of a pie. But that skinny sliver leaves you hungry and going back for another piece. You're back to one-sixth of the pie again—and that might leave your tummy groaning and overstuffed. But one-eighth of a pie is a satisfying, refreshing serving that will leave your palate happy!)

With Healthy Exchanges, those of you who are diabetic and hypoglycemic patients can find the "real world" desserts you've been missing. Again, while my own blood sugar is normal, both my parents and two uncles developed adult-onset diabetes. So creating delicious low-sugar recipes is a priority for me.

Live every day of your life as if you expected to live forever.

—Anonymous

Are you simply interested in preventing medical problems from developing? Are you ready to make a commitment to eat in a healthier way?

Maybe you're lucky enough to have no immediate medical concerns, but you would like to keep from developing them in the future. Perhaps you've seen all too clearly what the burdens of compromised health caused by a poor diet can be. You don't want to inherit the same "complications" you may have observed in parents and older family members, and you're determined to do your best to avoid future health problems by taking the necessary steps now. Healthy Exchanges will help you ensure lifelong good health.

Are you interested in quick and easy recipes the entire family will love?

Maybe you don't really care if a recipe is healthy or not. Maybe you have other priorities right now in your life, and you don't want to spend any more time than necessary in the kitchen. But because you and your family have to eat, you want a collection of good-tasting dishes that can be "thrown together" without much fuss. I will give you recipes for healthy, delicious food that often can be prepared in five minutes or less. (Not including unattended cooking time, but that time is freed for other projects!)

Did you answer "yes" to any of those questions? If you did, then **Healthy Exchanges** will give you just what you need—and deliciously, too!

I use your book daily. It has helped me lower my cholesterol from 400 to 225. . . . I've also lost weight.

—E. R., IA

Eat healthily, exercise moderately, think positively, and let those hips fall where they may!

Three

HELPing Yourself to Health

Nearly everyone I meet wants to know how I had the willpower to lose more than 130 pounds. They beg to hear my "secret"—and they're disappointed at first to hear that I don't have one. But perhaps it's fair to describe the HELP plan as a kind of treasure map—because it gets you where you want to go, and the end result is a real prize: good health.

Unlike a diet, which has a beginning and an end, the HELP plan is something you can live with for the rest of your life. And, if it's going to be the way you live now, you want to make the journey as pleasant as possible.

Let me tell you a little more about the four parts of HELP, the Healthy Exchanges Lifetime Plan—Healthy food, moderate Exercise, Lifetime changes, and Positive attitude. I'll be devoting an entire chapter to each of these a bit further on, but for now I'll give you a taste of what's to come—and some real-life evidence that HELP works!

HEALTHY EATING

Nothing tastes as good as thin feels.

You've already read about how I began to create healthy recipes, but here's the philosophy behind the healthy eating I prescribe. ***I make sure to treat myself well.***

If you don't believe what you've just read, ***read it again.*** Please.

By the time I made the decision to change the way I ate for the rest of my life, I'd eaten enough water-packed tuna on diet bread to last me a lifetime. I was always hungry afterward and too easily tempted to binge on donuts (my primary weakness!). I felt deprived, angry, and frustrated—and before I knew it, I was back devouring all the foods I'd told myself I wasn't "allowed" to touch. The result was a constant cycle of quick, brief weight loss followed by an even faster weight gain.

The secret of Healthy Exchanges, and the heart of the HELP program, is the recognition that we *need* to eat, that enjoyment is part of eating, and that we can no longer accept the social isolation of starvation diets that require us to eat a skimpy meal or drink a diet shake while our families and friends share a meal together.

Now I enjoy eating the foods I want, but I eat them in moderate quantities, and I create great-tasting healthy versions of foods I love—dishes that are low in fat and sugar.

No one said it better than in a letter I received a couple of years ago. Mary, a newsletter subscriber from Ohio, shared her success at losing more than sixty pounds with a national weight-loss support group. But, she wrote, "for the last six months, I have not been consistent, and I've gained back about twenty-five pounds. To put it bluntly, I had been fixing the same old standby dishes day in and day out and was bored with the routine."

She went on, "In the last few weeks I decided that I needed variety if I was going to live this way for the rest of my life. I knew that preparing my food differently and giving it some 'zip' was what it was all about. Your exciting new recipes that I have finally begun to prepare really have been the catalyst to help me succeed again."

But the best thing she told me was this: "I don't feel one bit deprived. As a matter of fact, I am so full eating your recipes I almost felt I would gain instead of losing weight. The portions seem very generous, and because I'm satisfied with my food now, I no longer desire the unhealthy foods that got me into trouble in the first place."

Mary, you're an inspiration to all of us!

What a difference it makes if we don't feel deprived! You did that, JoAnna, and how I thank you. May you continue to help those who want new ways.

—B. J., CO

MODERATE EXERCISE

I'm no fitness buff, but I know that I feel better when I include moderate exercise in my daily schedule. I'm probably the busiest person I know, so if I can make time for this, I'm confident you can, too—especially once you figure out what you enjoy doing, and then set a fitness goal. I discovered that my success in keeping this commitment was tied to making a game out of it, as I'll explain in chapter 5, but to pique your interest, I'll just say that every year I walk to New York (on paper!); every twelve months I ride my bike to Los Angeles; and I do water aerobics for a full week—well, not all in a row, but for a total of at least 168 hours!

Because I really enjoy my chosen exercises, I do them regularly and consider them my "fun." There are all kinds of scientific reasons that exercising makes us healthier, from increasing metabolism to burning calories and fat faster, to activating chemicals in the blood that increase our feeling of well-being. I read those reports in the newspaper, just as you do, but I also remember that next week there may be a new study that says something completely different. All I know is what I've learned from my own experience, and from others who have shared their feelings with me. *When I make time in my busy life to exercise regularly, I feel better about myself.* I have more energy, I don't seem to crave foods that aren't good for me, and I know it's helping me sustain the 130-pound weight loss that took me most of my life to accomplish.

If you've never exercised, I'll show you how to start slowly but surely to make it part of your life. If you used to exercise but now always seem to find excuses, I'll try to help you remember how good you feel when you do it.

And I won't let you off if you say you can't exercise because the weather's too bad. I'm from IOWA, remember? We get winters so snowy and windy, they practically knock you over! JoAnn, a woman I profiled in my newsletter, wrote that she enjoys walking and practicing line dancing in her basement during the bitter weather. "It's almost too much fun to be considered exercise," she told me. Well, just because something is fun doesn't mean it can't be good for you too!

A friend once recounted something that Dr. George Sheehan explained about exercise. When someone says, "The spirit is willing but the body is weak," *don't believe it*. The body is more than willing, but we need to give it a chance to feel as good as it possibly can. Our bodies are created with so much potential for good health, but too many of us lose sight of those wonderful possibilities.

As the popular athletic shoe ad says, "Just do it." You'll be more than pleased with the results.

If you want your dreams to come true, don't oversleep.

LIFETIME CHANGES

Do I hear you say you think you're too busy to follow the HELP plan? Too set in your ways? Hate to cook? Hate exercise? Never learned how to set a goal? Never believed you could reach one you set?

When you want something badly enough, you are granted the power to make it happen, but you have to be willing to make some changes in your life. Change can be scary, but the modest changes you'll be making in the way you live will have a positive effect on everything you do. It's not enough just to eat healthily, or just to exercise, or just to set a goal of better health, or just to think more positively about yourself. All these ingredients work together to help you reach your dream.

Everywhere you look, there are people offering you "easy" ways to lose pounds and pounds in one short week, or expensive exercise equipment that will give you a perfect body in ten minutes a day. Aren't you tired of all these promises that haven't been kept?

I want to show you how to make changes for a lifetime, ***one day at a time.*** Don't think about forever, or even about the months it may take you to reach your goals of losing so many pounds or lowering cholesterol so many points. We've been prisoners of the diet calendar for years, insisting that a program help us lose a set number of pounds in a specific length of time—or else we weren't interested. The result: discouraging failures, lowered self-esteem, and a sense of hopelessness.

Hope is wishing for a thing to come true; faith is believing that it will come true.

—Anonymous

I created HELP to offer another "four-letter word": HOPE. With hope, you'll be able to make changes for a lifetime, *lifetime* changes that will help you reach the health goals that once seemed so impossible and so far-off.

And don't think the only acceptable goals are serious ones, either. Patsy, from Arizona, told me she had four goals in mind for her fiftieth birthday:

1. To weigh 125 pounds. (She had only a couple of pounds to go . . .)
2. To renew her wedding vows on her twelfth anniversary.
3. To parachute from an airplane.
4. To perform onstage with a tap-dance group called The Hot Flashes.

What an amazing woman she is, moving full speed ahead into the second half of her life! Why not give yourself the best birthday present ever, just as Patsy did, by making a few of your fondest dreams real?

POSITIVE ATTITUDE

When I first began my HELP plan, I told myself: I will take it one day at a time. I will try to do the best I can—*the best I can*—for that twenty-four-hour period. Well, I'm still doing my best to live by that belief. I have good days when everything clicks and I think that living this way is the easiest thing I have ever done. But I'm human—I also have bad days when I eat more than I planned to. I have days when I wonder if it's worth the bother. Overall, though, I have more good days than bad ones because I want to eat healthier now than I did before, because I make an effort to fit exercise into my life, because I've made changes in my life to make the plan work, because I know I deserve to feel good about myself.

But everyone needs a reminder. Begin by saying to yourself every day: "From now on, I promise to be good to myself and to my family. I promise to get off the diet merry-go-round. I promise to enjoy life!"

There, doesn't that feel good? If you hear those promises aloud, they start to become real. They start to become possible. Listen to yourself, and listen to your heart. You'll be HELPing yourself become the best you can be.

When people come to hear me, they're often looking for someone to help them get started. When I tell them there's no magic anything in what I do, that there's just my daily routine, sometimes they look disappointed. But I go on to say that it doesn't require magic—just patience, a willingness to make changes in your life, and a commitment to live better from this moment on.

As the old saying goes, Rome wasn't built in a day. Anything important takes time, but the time is going to pass anyway. Why not do something good for yourself *today?* Make no mistake, though. I'm no Pollyanna, but I do try to look at things in the best possible light. After all, it helps you get through the day.

And when I may be wavering a bit (I'm human; I keep telling you that!), I find myself uplifted by the stories shared by members of the Healthy Exchanges family. One who won my heart was Norman, from New Hampshire, who reminded me that you must examine all that you have accomplished, instead of focusing on one bad day or week. "Look at where you are now," he said, "and don't let yourself slide back to where you were. Instead of bad-mouthing yourself, congratulate yourself for whatever you've done in a positive way. Maybe you took a ten-minute walk today instead of collapsing on the couch." He added, "Don't forget that even if you only lost one-half pound this month, that's still two sticks of butter you're not wearing anymore!"

I hope this will be the answer to my prayers.

—J. D., IN

There you have the four parts of HELP, in brief. In the next four chapters, I'll give you all you need to know to live the HELP lifestyle, and to *succeed,* especially if you feel you're looking back on a history of failure.

Why does HELP work? I think because it encompasses every aspect of living. I don't zero in on just calling this a diet, and I'm not coming at you from the exercise/fitness side, saying, "Work out, and it's all going to fall into place." I'm not suggesting that your only problem is figuring out what goals to set. And I'm not saying

South St. Paul Public Library
106 Third Avenue North
South St. Paul, MN 55075

My purpose in trying Healthy Exchanges was to lower my cholesterol. Well, mission accomplished! I had my yearly physical this week, and it had gone from 262 to 203.

—D. L., AZ

you have to understand behavior modification to solve your problems.

What I am saying is work with me on the surface on all these areas, and we will eventually work down to why.

In the meantime, we are already working on a solution. I think you can start to become stronger *before* you face the underlying causes. Think of this behavior as "acting as if," even if you're not ready yet. "Dress for Success"—even if you don't have the job yet. Start living healthily immediately—even if you're not healthy yet. And pretty soon, you will be.

HELP WORKS!

In case it's not enough that *I* keep telling you that HELP works, and that it will work for you, let me share some of the chorus of support that sustains me on a daily basis:

From Roy, who's had six heart bypasses:

"I have recovered and feel great. Your recipes are fantastic for meals and out of this world for desserts. I volunteer at the hospital where I had the surgery doing what we call our Heart to Heart program. We give the family support during the operation, and also visit the heart patients in their rooms. When people tell me they're worried about preparing good healthy meals, I just give them the address for Healthy Exchanges."

From Amy, a young mother with diabetes who uses an insulin pump:

"I've been a diabetic for twelve years and count carbohydrates in order to figure my insulin dosages. I use the carbohydrate counts more than the diabetic exchanges, but I'm glad to have both." Amy told me she is looking forward to getting pregnant with a second child, especially since she won't have to exist on boring snacks and meals again, as she did in her first pregnancy. "I used to pack a cooler every day for work with all my little items to eat for snacks and meals throughout the day. I needed to eat six meals a day to obtain a nice level and low blood sugar. I used to eat the same thing every day. It'll be easier the second time with JoAnna's recipes."

It's never too late to try and live healthy.

—B. B., NH

From Jo, an eighty-two-year-old widow:

"I like the easy, quick recipes and especially that they are within the budget of one on a fixed income. . . . My doctor is very pleased with my cholesterol count too. Healthy Exchanges is great to live with!"

From Maxine, a seventy-year-old grandmother:

I have lost 133 pounds since a year ago last April. I want to lose 17 more pounds. My kids tell me I'm not the same person anymore. . . . I know I feel better than I have for forty years. . . . My kids tell me I sure don't look seventy and I sure don't feel it."

Be not afraid of growing slowly, be only afraid of standing still.

—Chinese proverb

And finally, Melinda, a teacher from Michigan, who's living proof of HELP's potential:

She counts fat grams and has lost at least fifty pounds, although she doesn't weigh herself anymore. She lets her clothing do the measuring for her. Melinda went from a snug size 20 to a slim size 10. She even bought a few size 8s recently.

"Just make a start in your new healthy lifestyle," Melinda says. "The start doesn't have to be huge. Set small, attainable goals. And don't wait until you think you know everything about healthy living. You will learn as you go. Last but not least, *don't be in a hurry.* You'll be doing this for the rest of your life, so enjoy every day."

Ready to feel good, look better, become healthier than you ever have in your life? *All right!* Come with me, and I'll give you the tools you'll need to start incorporating HELP into your life.

Part Two

THE FOUR PARTS OF HELP

By eating the Healthy Exchanges way, I'm happy to report I lost weight. I'm going on seventy-nine, I feel great, and am full of pep most of the time.

—H. S., OH

Four

Healthy Exchanges Eating: How It Works

Let's eat!

But wait, do I detect a lack of enthusiasm here?

Do you, like most dieters, and others who have decided to eat low-fat and low-sugar meals, expect that your pleasure in eating will be diminished? Are you convinced that healthy cooking will be bland, boring, and predictable, contain few of the foods you really enjoy, and offer tiny portions that wouldn't satisfy a child?

Well, Healthy Exchanges will change all that—from the first recipe you prepare and the first meal you share with your family!

I learned how to eat well—without sacrificing my health—when I finally understood that part of living a healthy lifestyle is creating meals you and your family will be able to enjoy together. It's no coincidence that the first healthy recipe I created was Mexicalli Pie, a spicy, meaty hearty main dish I knew would pass the Cliff Lund Taste Test. Before I ever went into the kitchen, I asked myself, "What kinds of food does my husband like best?" I wanted to sit down to healthy meals that we could *share*—so they had to be delicious enough to appeal to everyone.

Healthy Exchanges food fills you up without filling you out.

When Low-Fat Is Too Low

If you think your family, or anyone else, will voluntarily eat something just because "it's good for them," think again! Sure, you can find main-dish recipes that have only one or two grams of fat per serving, and yes, there are desserts that are totally sugar free. But do you and your loved ones find them tasty enough to enjoy again and again? The most important principle to lifelong healthy eating is that if you want people to eat "what's good for them," you have to prepare what *tastes* good to them, too.

Food has to please both our bodies and souls. Each of us has different comfort foods from childhood, different tastes that make us feel good inside. Maybe we can't or we shouldn't have the high-fat, high-sugar versions we recall with such pleasure—but we can stir up dishes that duplicate the same textures, flavors, and aromas.

This might mean enjoying a main dish that clocks in at eight grams of fat per serving instead of the original twenty-five grams or more. Yes, it's possible to prepare versions that are practically fat free, but if they don't deliver enough flavor to satisfy us, we won't eat them again. My "common folk," healthy recipes are designed to be a bridge between those high-fat dishes that no longer fit into a healthy lifestyle and the currently popular but often tasteless fat-free and sugar-free recipes.

Learning What Makes Healthy Exchanges Work

I'm often asked, "Just tell me what you do so I can do the same." I think you'll find that Healthy Exchanges eating is not about what I

I made a broccoli cheese dish that called for cream of broccoli soup. Well, I didn't have that, so used cream of mushroom. And it called for broccoli but all I had in the house was cauliflower. So when my family asked what it was, I said broccoli cheese something. . . . They couldn't find the broccoli and decided I was nuts . . . but it's a great example of using the recipes simply as a road map—the variation is up to us.

—P. P., MI

do—*it's about doing what will work for you*, and for the rest of your life. I'm definitely not a believer in a cookie-cutter approach to healthy living. Diet plans that dictate everyone should eat grapefruit for breakfast each Tuesday morning have never worked for me—and they probably haven't worked for you, either. Most of us like the freedom to choose. We want to be able to choose *this* instead of that, and we feel resentful if someone restricts our choices. That's why most diets fail—we get tired of the regimentation, and we're not satisfied by what we eat.

Once you learn to use the Healthy Exchanges Choice/Exchange system, you'll have the tools you need to create your own versions of favorite foods.

Here's how the system works. Foods are divided into basic food groups and portion sizes determined so that all contain approximately the same nutritional values. These groups include Proteins/Meats, Breads/Starches, Vegetables, Fats, Fruits, Skim Milk, Free Foods, and Optional Calories. While the Weight Loss Choices and the Diabetic Exchanges are similar, there are important differences. This is why I've provided both for you, in addition to listing calories, fat and fiber grams, protein grams, carbohydrate grams, and sodium.

Each food choice included in a particular group has about the same calories, carbohydrates, protein, and fat content as all the others. You can "exchange" one choice for another, and as long as you select the right number of choices in each group each day, you'll be eating healthy foods and in reasonable portions.

Here's an example: bread, pasta, and corn are choices in the Bread/Starches group. One choice or exchange lets you choose 1 slice of bread, *or* ½ cup of cooked pasta, *or* ½ cup corn. You've got a variety of foods to choose from in each category, and *you* don't have to calculate the nutrient values—it's already been done for you! In the pages that follow, I'll explain which foods fit into which group, and how to figure the right quantities to eat. You can cook for one, or for a crowd, and still know exactly how many portions—"choices"—in each group you've used.

I don't want to make it seem as if my recipes are the only way to make Healthy Exchanges eating work. Try thinking of them as a kind of road map on your journey to better health, and remember that you're free to take side trips to fit your family's likes and dislikes. My menu suggestions are just that—*suggestions*—that I designed to show you just how well you can eat, and how to use a variety of ingredients to make your healthy meals appealing and delicious. If you don't feel like serving Easy Lasagna on the designated evening, choose another main dish that you like better. (You won't hurt my feelings—I promise!)

What's important is that you don't have to eat what you don't like anymore. Feel free to eliminate mushrooms if your family can't stomach them, or switch asparagus for green beans if it's more to your taste. Just don't tamper with the basic integrity of the recipe, so you'll get the full flavor and appearance of each good-tasting dish.

What about Calories and Fats?

No matter what you may have heard from other sources about what an acceptable percent of calories from fat may be, or how many calories you can or should be consuming, I'm here to tell you that *calories do count.* Some programs claim that as long as you keep your fat calories below a certain level, you can eat all you want—but I disagree, and common sense backs me up.

If your body only requires 1,600 calories a day to lose weight at a moderate rate, and about 2,100 calories to maintain your weight, what do you think happens if you're consuming only 10 grams of fat but eating 5,000 calories a day to feel satisfied? Your body can't use the excess, and you're going to gain weight instead of losing it.

The sample menus I've created provide about 1,600 calories per day, and my Weight Loss Choices/Exchanges, calories-from-fat percentage, and Diabetic Exchanges are based on this figure. This should be enough to keep your tummy satisfied and still allow you to lose weight gradually.

You'll notice I don't worry about a hard-and-fast number when it comes to figuring an allowable percentage of calories from fat. We know that most Americans include far too much fat in their diets—some as much as 40 to 50 percent of a day's calories! In my suggested Healthy Exchanges menus, the percentage of calories from fat will range from a low of 15 percent to a high of about 25 percent. But the overall weekly rate will average out to about 20

I have reached my goal weight! It has taken me nine and a half months to attain this state of nirvana in which my total weight loss to date has been forty-four pounds. I would not have been as successful as this without the help and encouragement of your recipes. Thank you! Your concept of weight loss through learning to eat properly makes the whole process easier to follow.

—A.O., IA

You can't eat what you don't buy.

percent of calories derived from fat—enough to keep you healthy and satisfied, while you still lose weight.

Remember this: *Too much of anything is still too much*—no matter how good it is for you! Don't fall into the trap of overeating high-volume, low-fat foods. It is very possible to gain weight—even if you are consuming fewer than 15 grams of fat and very little processed sugar each day. If your body requires a certain number of calories, and you regularly eat 1,000 a day more, those excess calories must be deposited somewhere.

(Just my luck—those critters always seemed to congregate around my hips and carry on a convention!)

So please don't think that just because those bakery treats or ice cream products are marked "fat-free" and "sugar-free," you can enjoy them to your heart's content. Trust me, your heart won't be all that happy with you—and neither will your waistline!

Nothing in life is truly free, and so it is with the food we eat. Fat-free products are a boon to those of us who want to lose weight and lower our cholesterol, but they are in no way a license to overindulge. Just take a good look at the ingredients and calories per serving on that box of pastry treats marked "fat-free." You may be surprised to see how high in sugar and calories they are! An occasional serving is fine, but eating the entire box of goodies isn't. *Moderation* is the key.

The same holds true for sugar-free products. How many people have you overheard at fast-food restaurants ordering a diet soda—and french fries?

There's no magic answer, but I think I've come pretty close to the solution. I've quit fooling myself by abusing fat-free and sugar-free products. I use them in moderation in my recipes, incorporating them into my healthy lifestyle. But I know my hips and my health will pay the price if I overdo it.

Instead, I enjoy an abundant variety of foods prepared in flavorful ways. I like to say that Healthy Exchanges food "fills you *up* without filling you *out!*"

Determining Actual Calorie Needs

There are a number of ways to determine calorie needs. They are based on a person's weight, actual or desirable, plus height and activity levels. None of them is perfect, but they can give you some guidance in determining what your calorie intake level should be to help you lose or maintain weight.

The traditional rule for estimating desirable body weight:

Build	Adult Women	Adult Men
Medium	*100 pounds for the first five feet in height*	*106 pounds for the first five feet in height*
	Add 5 pounds for each inch over five feet	*Add 6 pounds for each inch over five feet*

If you have a small frame, subtract 10%; if you have a large frame, add 10%.

These are estimates, and they may not be right for you. Some authorities suggest a range of desirable weights. For example, one national weight-loss support group suggests that a woman who is 5′4″ should weigh 118 to 135 pounds.

See tables 1 and 2 for calorie and fat gram recommendations for your weight. Subtracting 500 to 1,000 calories per day usually leads to a 1- to 3-pound weight loss per week. Of course, there are many variables that will affect how a person loses weight, and adjustments often have to be made. Eating fewer than 1,200 calories per day is not advised and may lead to a decreased metabolic rate that slows the body's ability to burn calories.

TABLE 1

Recommendations for Men and Physically Active Women under Age 45

Weight *(desirable pounds)*	Maintenance Calories* *(x 15 calories/ pound)*	Calories from Fat†			
		15%	*20%*	*25%*	*30%*
		Women			
100	1,500	25g	35g	40g	50g
110	1,650	30g	35g	45g	55g
120	1,800	30g	40g	50g	60g
130	1,950	35g	45g	55g	65g
140	2,100	35g	45g	60g	70g
150	2,250	40g	50g	65g	75g
160	2,400	40g	55g	65g	80g
170	2,550	40g	55g	70g	85g
180	2,700	45g	60g	75g	90g
		Men			
135	2,025	35g	45g	55g	65g
145	2,175	35g	50g	60g	70g
155	2,325	40g	50g	65g	80g
165	2,475	40g	55g	70g	85g
175	2,625	45g	60g	75g	90g
185	2,775	45g	60g	75g	90g
195	2,925	50g	65g	80g	100g
205	3,075	50g	70g	85g	105g

* To lose weight, subtract 500 calories per day.
† Fat grams are rounded to nearest increment of 5.

Table prepared by Rose Hoenig, R.D., L.D.

TABLE 2

Recommendations for People over Age 45 or People Who Are Inactive

Weight (desirable pounds)	Maintenance Calories* (x 13 calories/ pound)	Calories from Fat†			
		15%	20%	25%	30%
		Women			
100	1,300	20g	30g	35g	45g
110	1,430	25g	30g	40g	50g
120	1,560	25g	35g	45g	50g
130	1,690	30g	40g	45g	55g
140	1,820	30g	40g	50g	60g
150	1,950	35g	45g	55g	65g
160	2,080	35g	45g	60g	70g
170	2,210	35g	50g	60g	75g
180	2,340	40g	50g	65g	80g
		Men			
135	1,755	30g	40g	50g	60g
145	1,885	30g	40g	50g	60g
155	2,015	35g	45g	55g	65g
165	2,145	35g	50g	60g	70g
175	2,275	40g	50g	65g	75g
185	2,405	40g	55g	65g	80g
195	2,535	40g	55g	70g	85g
205	2,665	45g	60g	75g	90g

* To lose weight, subtract 500 calories per day. If you eat fewer than 1,200 calories per day, a multivitamin/mineral supplement is recommended.
† Fat grams are rounded to nearest increment of 5.

Table prepared by Rose Hoenig, R.D., L.D.

Finding Out What Works for You

My niece gave me your newsletter as a gift after my husband had a heart attack last July. It has been the most-looked-forward-to piece of mail we get. It hasn't only benefited him but me as well. I have diabetes and have dropped my medication in half with the use of your recipes. They have really helped.

—L. S., LA

Everyone has a different lifestyle, and it's important to make Healthy Eating fit your schedule, instead of the other way around. My motto is **"Healthy lifestyle choices are like panty hose—one size does not fit all!"**

My largest meal is usually lunch, because I work at home and can plan around it. But because most people work full-time outside the home, I've planned the menus with dinner as the largest meal of the day.

Suppose you want to make dinner your main meal three days a week and lunch the biggest meal on the other days. *Do it!* Whatever works for you and your family is what makes sense.

When I first began eating the Healthy Exchanges way, my toughest time was always around 4:30 in the afternoon. No matter what I ate for lunch, I was always hungry then. (I believe part of it was habit, and part of it was my body's metabolism.) Before Healthy Exchanges, I would find myself eating one supper as I was fixing the "real" supper. But now that need to eat something could be handled as part of my healthy eating plan.

Every day at 4:30, when I got home from work, I fixed myself a healthy snack, sat down in my chair, and just enjoyed it. Sometimes I might turn the TV on, sometimes I might read the newspaper, sometimes I'd just sit there. I took that private time for me to connect with myself and enjoy that snack. By understanding what I needed, and when I needed it, I was able to nourish myself the right way. (You'll see that my sample menus include *two snacks* each day.)

But just because I want you to do what works for you does NOT give you permission to eat ice cream three times a day and then have it again for a snack! You know when you are selecting a reasonable, healthy choice—and when you are rationalizing a bad habit back into your lifestyle.

Be careful not to tell yourself your goal is to lose the weight as fast as possible. That's *dieting*—and you're not going to do that anymore. Instead, tell yourself you're going to lose it at a slow, steady rate, and improve your chances of keeping it off forever. Because you're taking the time to develop good, healthy habits, you're going to succeed this time.

Tracking Your New Healthy Lifestyle

Keeping track of the servings you eat each day will help you stay focused—and make sure you're enjoying all the food you're "entitled" to.

I've included a sample Healthy Exchanges Weight Loss Choices Daily Planner, which shows you how to keep track of your daily exchanges. I've also supplied a list of choices for each type of exchange. For each food group, there are places to cross out the choices/exchanges (or fractions thereof) that you've eaten, so you'll always know what you have left to enjoy—and so you can plan your day.

If, at the end of the day, they're not accounted for 100 percent, don't worry that you'll have to sit up past midnight finishing your quarter of a Fruit or third of a Protein exchange! I don't expect you to take two bites of an apple and throw it out. *Let's get real.* Nothing in life comes out exactly as planned—but you do the best you can.

Starting on page 66 I've shown a Daily Planner completed from breakfast through lunch, dinner, and two snacks. Follow this easy example if you're confused about record keeping. I've also included separate daily planners if your choice is to count calories, fat, and fiber grams, or to count Diabetic Exchanges.

I personally figure the Weight Loss Choices, I use the Food Processor II software to calculate calories and grams, and registered dietitian Rose Hoenig figures the Diabetic Exchanges.

(I think I could do the Weight Loss Choices in my sleep. My son Tommy once remarked that the food values of the ingredients I use are to me what baseball statistics are to him!)

I was recently diagnosed a diabetic and have been following a closely prescribed program but find the inclusion of your unique recipes a great treat. "Hats off" to you, JoAnna, for your creative talents and for sharing them with so many.

—A. P., AZ

WHAT ABOUT SUBSTITUTIONS?

Whenever I give two options, such as one egg *or* the equivalent in egg substitute, the first ingredient listed is the one used in the calculations. If you chose to use egg substitute instead, your actual fat gram count would be even less than that shown for the recipe. I can hear some people asking, "If the egg substitute is lower in fat, why don't you use just that?"

I don't play the "numbers" game as some recipe developers do. I create the recipe first and then do the calculations, not the other way around. I also ask myself how most of the people who live in "the real world" would prepare the recipe. When I cook for myself and my family, I don't want to spend the money on egg substitute, and I don't want to spend the extra time dividing yolks from whites. Instead, I choose to limit my egg consumption to four eggs a week, and enjoy them in baked products or salad much more than in a fried-egg sandwich, for example.

For anyone who *must* limit egg consumption even more than this for medical reasons, I test the recipe using both "real" eggs and egg substitute. I do the same for every recipe that gives you more than one option. This is my responsibility when I am wearing my Healthy Exchanges chef's hat—and I don't share a recipe that offers an option until I know the result is delicious both ways.

Remember, due to the inevitable variations in the ingredients you choose to use because of availability or personal taste, the nutritional values should be considered approximate.

Sliders are part of the plan. They are designed to be used on a daily basis—to give you flexibility, to satisfy hunger, and to provide you with options to live your life. If you "use up" your two Skim Milk exchanges but your planned snack includes another skim milk serving, enjoy! It's good for you, and all you need to do is check off one of your Sliders. If you've already used your Sliders for the day, then make a withdrawal from your bank of Optional Calories. Each Slider equals approximately 80 calories.

HELP is a Lifetime Plan. I chose those words on purpose, to help you begin to see how you can make healthy eating choices for the rest of your life. Some days, you may find that you're completely satisfied by the regular exchanges and use only a modest number of Optional Calories and/or Sliders. Other days, you may

Healthy Exchanges Weight Loss Choices™ or Exchanges Daily Planner

Day: ______________________________

Skim Milk	¼	⅓	½	⅔	¾	1		¼	⅓	½	⅔	¾	1
Fat	¼	⅓	½	⅔	¾	1		¼	⅓	½	⅔	¾	1
Fruit	¼	⅓	½	⅔	¾	1		¼	⅓	½	⅔	¾	1
	¼	⅓	½	⅔	¾	1							
Vegetable	¼	⅓	½	⅔	¾	1		¼	⅓	½	⅔	¾	1
	¼	⅓	½	⅔	¾	1		¼	⅓	½	⅔	¾	1
Protein	¼	⅓	½	⅔	¾	1		¼	⅓	½	⅔	¾	1
	¼	⅓	½	⅔	¾	1		¼	⅓	½	⅔	¾	1
	¼	⅓	½	⅔	¾	1							
Bread	¼	⅓	½	⅔	¾	1		¼	⅓	½	⅔	¾	1
	¼	⅓	½	⅔	¾	1		¼	⅓	½	⅔	¾	1
	¼	⅓	½	⅔	¾	1							
Slider	¼	⅓	½	⅔	¾	1		¼	⅓	½	⅔	¾	1
	¼	⅓	½	⅔	¾	1		¼	⅓	½	⅔	¾	1

Optional Calories	10	20	30	40	50	60	70	80	90	100

Water

Vitamin

Remember, if you require more or fewer selections because of your personal needs, adjust your daily intake accordingly. This chart is intended to be only a guide in helping you count your daily selections. After using your Skim Milk, Fruit, Protein, or Bread selections for the day, use additional choices for these in the Slider.

For me, cancer was a wake-up call. For the first time, I started relating my weight—and what I eat—to staying alive. I've always been an emotional eater, and I lied to myself a lot over the years. Now it's time to do it right.

—N. B., ND

choose to use everything on your Planner, or *even run a few calories over.* That's my point. This is real life, not a diet.

If you choose not to count Weight Loss Choices/exchanges, Healthy Exchanges recipes still provide an abundance of helpful nutritional information that can assist you in living a healthy lifestyle. Many people, particularly those interested in lowering or controlling their cholesterol, decide to track their fat grams on a daily basis. Some like to add up fiber or carbohydrate grams, while others prefer to count the calories in the dishes they enjoy.

Here's a planner that will give you a place to record your daily calorie and fat and fiber gram counts. The daily Healthy Exchanges menus I've created provide an average of 1,600 calories per day (with approximately 20 percent of calories coming from fat). These menus average 35 grams of fat and 20 grams of fiber, although you'll see that the chart provides room for additional grams *as needed.* Suggested guidelines for fat and fiber consumption do vary, so please check with a physician or nutrition professional if you have questions about what number of grams is best for you.

I've also included a Diabetic Exchanges diary, because so many diabetics have found Healthy Exchanges recipes a perfect fit for their doctor-recommended diabetic diets. This planner was designed in consultation with health-care professionals and provides boxes to check off standard diabetic exchanges: 2 Skim Milk, 3 Fat, up to 8 Vegetable, 5 Meat, up to 10 Starch, as well as room to track Free Food and Carbohydrates. Consider these *as a guideline only*, as your medical provider will determine the appropriate number of daily exchanges and carbohydrate grams for you.

Healthy Exchanges Calories with Fat and Fiber Gram Counter

Day: _____ Daily allowance average of 1,600 calories with 35 fat grams or about 20% of calories coming from fat and about 20 fiber grams

Breakfast	calories _________	fat grams _________	fiber grams _________
Lunch	calories _________	fat grams _________	fiber grams _________
Dinner	calories _________	fat grams _________	fiber grams _________
Snack(s)	calories _________	fat grams _________	fiber grams _________
	calories _________	fat grams _________	fiber grams _________
Daily Total	calories _________	fat grams _________	fiber grams _________

Add more grams if needed for your daily requirements.

Daily Fat Gram Counter

1	2	3	4	5	6	7	8	9	10	11	12	13	14	15	16	17	18	19	20
21	22	23	24	25	26	27	28	29	30	31	32	33	34	35	36	37	38	39	
40	41	42	43	44	45	46	47	48	49	50	51	52	53	54	55	56	57	58	59	60

Daily Fiber Gram Counter

1	2	3	4	5	6	7	8	9	10	11	12	13	14	15	16	17	18	19	20	
21	22	23	24	25	26	27	28	29	30	31	32	33	34	35	36	37	38	39		
40	41	42	43	44	45	46	47	48	49	50	51	52	53	54	55	56	57	58	59	60

Remember, if you require more or fewer calories because of your individual needs, adjust your daily intake accordingly. Just try to average about 20% of your calories coming from fat and at least 15 to 20 fiber grams each day. This chart is intended to be only a guide in helping you count your daily calories and fat and fiber grams.

Healthy Exchanges Diabetic Exchanges Diary

Day:__________

Breakfast A.M. Snack Lunch P.M. Snack Dinner Evening Snack

Skim Milk

½	½	½	½

Fat

½	½	½	½
½	½		

Fruit

½	½	½	½
½	½	½	½

Vegetable

½	½	½	½
½	½	½	½
½	½	½	½
½	½	½	½

Meat

½	½	½	½
½	½	½	½
½	½		

Starch

½	½	½	½
½	½	½	½
½	½	½	½
½	½	½	½
½	½	½	½

Free Food

½	½	½	½

Carbohydrate Tracker

5 10 15 20 25 30 35 40 45 50 55 60 65 70 75 80 85 90 95 100
105 110 115 120 125 130 135 140 145 150 155 160 165 170 175
180 185 190 195 200 205 210 215 220 225 230 235 240 245 250 255 260

The sole purpose of this chart is to provide an average of daily diabetic exchanges based on 1,600 calories per day. ADD or DELETE exchanges as your health-care provider recommends. All diabetics should have their own personal daily exchanges and carbohydrate intake determined by their medical providers.

Healthy Exchanges Weight Loss Choices/Exchanges

If you've ever been on one of the national weight-loss programs like Weight Watchers or Diet Center, you've already been introduced to the concept of measured portions of different food groups that make up your daily food plan. If you are not familiar with such a system of weight-loss choices or exchanges, here's a brief explanation. (If you want or need more detailed information, you can write to the American Dietetic Association* or the American Diabetes Association† for comprehensive explanations.)

The idea of food exchanges is to divide foods into basic food groups. The foods in each group are measured in servings that have comparable values. These groups include Proteins/Meats, Breads/Starches, Vegetables, Fats, Fruits, Skim Milk, Free Foods, and Optional Calorics.

Each choice or exchange included in a particular group has about the same number of calories and a similar carbohydrate, protein, and fat content as the other foods in that group. Because any food on a particular list can be "exchanged" for any other food in that group, it makes sense to call the food groups *exchanges* or *choices*.

I like to think we are also "exchanging" bad habits and food choices for good ones!

By using Weight Loss Choices or exchanges you can choose from a variety of foods without having to calculate the nutrient value of each one. This makes it easier to include a wide variety of foods in your daily menus and gives you the opportunity to tailor your choices to your unique appetite.

If you want to lose weight, you should consult your physician or other weight-control expert regarding the number of servings that would be best for you from each food group. Since men generally require more calories than women, and since the requirements for growing children and teenagers differ from those for

* 1225 I Street NW, Washington, D.C. 20005
† 1211 Connecticut Avenue NW, Washington, D.C. 20036

adults, the right number of exchanges for any one person is a personal decision.

I have included a suggested plan of Weight Loss Choices in the pages following the exchange lists. It's a program I used to lose 130 pounds, and it's the one I still follow today.

Because not everyone wants or needs to lose weight with Healthy Exchanges, I've also provided a planner to help you count fat and fiber grams, and one for tracking Diabetic Exchanges. For a brief explanation of how they are used, turn to page 49.

(If you are a diabetic or have been diagnosed with heart problems, it is best to meet with your physician before using this or any other food program or recipe collection.)

FOOD GROUP EXCHANGES

Proteins

Meat, poultry, seafood, eggs, cheese, and legumes. One exchange of Protein is approximately 60 calories. Examples of one Protein choice or exchange:

1 ounce cooked weight of lean meat, poultry, or seafood
2 ounces white fish
1½ ounces 97% fat-free ham
1 egg (limit to no more than 4 per week)
¼ cup egg substitute
3 egg whites
¾ ounce reduced-fat cheese
½ cup fat-free cottage cheese
2 ounces cooked or ¾ ounces uncooked dry beans
1 tablespoon peanut butter (also count 1 fat exchange)

Breads

Breads, crackers, cereals, grains, and starchy vegetables. One exchange of Bread is approximately 80 calories. Examples of one Bread choice or exchange:

1 slice bread or 2 slices reduced-calorie bread (40 calories or less)
1 roll, any type (1 ounce)
½ cup cooked pasta or ¾ ounce uncooked (scant ½ cup)
½ cup cooked rice or 1 ounce uncooked (⅓ cup)
3 tablespoons flour
¾ ounce cold cereal
½ cup cooked hot cereal or ¾ ounce uncooked (2 tablespoons)
½ cup corn (kernels or cream style) or peas
4 ounces white potato, cooked, or 5 ounces uncooked
3 ounces sweet potato, cooked, or 4 ounces uncooked
3 cups air-popped popcorn
7 fat-free crackers (¾ ounce)
3 (2½-inch squares) graham crackers
2 (¾-ounce) rice cakes or 6 mini
1 tortilla, any type (6-inch diameter)

Fruits

All fruits and fruit juices. One exchange of Fruit is approximately 60 calories. Examples of one Fruit choice or exchange:

1 small apple or ½ cup slices
1 small orange
½ medium banana
¾ cup berries (except strawberries and cranberries)
1 cup strawberries or cranberries
½ cup canned fruit, packed in fruit juice or rinsed well
2 tablespoons raisins
1 tablespoon spreadable fruit spread
½ cup apple juice (4 fluid ounces)
½ cup orange juice (4 fluid ounces)
½ cup applesauce

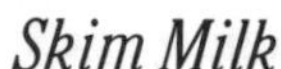

Skim Milk

Milk, buttermilk, and yogurt. One exchange of Skim Milk is approximately 90 calories. Examples of one Skim Milk choice or exchange:

1 cup skim milk
½ cup evaporated skim milk
1 cup low-fat buttermilk
¾ cup plain fat-free yogurt
⅓ cup nonfat dry milk powder

Vegetables

All fresh, canned, or frozen vegetables other than the starchy vegetables. One exchange of Vegetable is approximately 30 calories. Examples of one Vegetable choice or exchange:

½ cup vegetable
¼ cup tomato sauce
1 medium fresh tomato
½ cup vegetable juice

Fats

Margarine, mayonnaise, vegetable oils, salad dressings, olives, and nuts. One exchange of fat is approximately 40 calories. Examples of one Fat choice or exchange:

1 teaspoon margarine or 2 teaspoons reduced-calorie margarine
1 teaspoon butter
1 teaspoon vegetable oil
1 teaspoon mayonnaise or 2 teaspoons reduced-calorie mayonnaise
1 teaspoon peanut butter
1 ounce olives
¼ ounce pecans, walnuts, peanuts, or pistachios

Free Foods

Foods that do not provide nutritional value but are used to enhance the taste of foods are included in the Free Foods group. Examples of these are spices, herbs, extracts, vinegar, lemon juice, mustard, Worcestershire sauce, and soy sauce. Cooking sprays and artificial sweeteners used in moderation are also included in this group. However, you'll see that I include the caloric value of artificial sweeteners in the Optional Calories of the recipes.

You may occasionally see a recipe that lists "free food" as part of the portion. According to the published exchange lists, a free food contains fewer than 20 calories per serving. Two or three servings per day of free foods/drinks are usually allowed in a meal plan.

Optional Calories

Foods that do not fit into any other group but are used in moderation in recipes are included in Optional Calories. Foods that are counted in this way include sugar-free gelatin and puddings, fat-free mayonnaise and dressings, reduced-calorie whipped toppings, reduced-calorie syrups and jams, chocolate chips, coconut, and canned broth.

Sliders™

These are eighty Optional Calorie increments that do not fit into any particular category. You can choose which food group to *slide* them into. It is wise to limit this selection to approximately three per day to ensure the best possible nutrition for your body while still enjoying an occasional treat.

Sliders™ may be used in either of the following ways:

1. If you have consumed all your Protein (Pr), Bread (Br), Fruit (Fr), or Skim Milk (SM) Weight Loss Choices for the day and you want to eat additional foods from those food groups, you simply use a Slider (Sl). It's what I call "healthy horse trading."

I'm the seventy-year-old lady who wrote you a while back. I have lost the rest of my weight, so I've lost 150 pounds in a year and a half and feel like I'm thirty again.

I'm a retired nurse's aide living in Illinois and taking care of my aunt (eighty-one and with Alzheimer's) and my uncle (seventy-four and has emphysema). They love your pies! I make one every day. I have made twenty-four different pies and they are all delicious. The whole neighborhood knows about your pies and nobody will believe they're diet pies. But I'm living proof. I ate a piece of every one of them and haven't gained a pound.

—M. H., IL

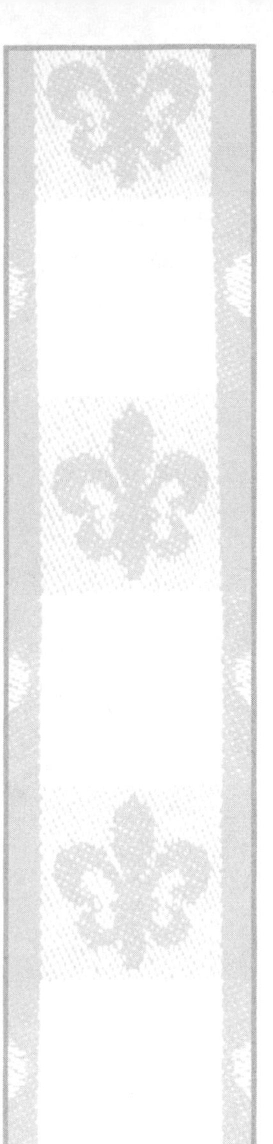

2. Sliders may also be deducted from your Optional Calories (OC) for the day or week. ¼ Sl equals 20 OC; ½ Sl equals 40 OC; ¾ Sl equals 60 OC; and 1 Sl equals 80 OC. This way, you can choose the food group to *slide* them into.

A word about Sliders: These are to be counted toward your totals after you have used your allotment of choices of Skim Milk, Protein, Bread, and Fruit for the day. By "sliding" an additional choice into one of these groups, you can meet your individual needs for that day. Sliders are especially helpful when traveling, stressed-out, eating out, or for special events. I often use mine so I can enjoy my favorite Healthy Exchanges desserts. Vegetables are not to be counted as Sliders. Enjoy as many Vegetable Choices as you need to feel satisfied. Because we want to limit our fat intake to moderate amounts, additional Fat Choices should not be counted as Sliders. If you choose to include more fat on an *occasional* basis, count the extra choices as Optional Calories.

HEALTHY EXCHANGES® WEIGHT LOSS CHOICES™

Here's my suggested program of Weight Loss Choices for women, based on an average daily total of 1,400 to 1,600 calories per day. *If you require more or fewer calories, please revise this plan to your individual needs.*

Each day, you should plan to eat:

2 Skim Milk (SM) servings, 90 calories each
2 Fat (Fa) servings, 40 calories each
3 Fruit (Fr) servings, 60 calories each
4 Vegetable (Ve) servings or more, 30 calories each
5 Protein (Pr) servings, 60 calories each
5 Bread (Br) servings, 80 calories each

You may also choose to add up to 100 Optional Calories per day, and up to 28 Sliders per week at 80 calories each. If you choose to include more Sliders in your daily or weekly totals, deduct those 80 calories from your Optional Calorie "bank."

Keep a daily food diary of your Weight Loss Choices, checking off what you eat as you go. If, at the end of the day, your required selections are not 100 percent accounted for, but you have done the best you can, go to bed with a clear conscience. There will be days when you have ¼ Fruit or ½ Bread left over. What are you going to do—eat two slices of an orange or half a slice of bread and throw the rest out? I always say that "nothing in life comes out exactly." Just do the best you can . . . *the best you can.*

Try to drink at least 8 glasses of water a day. Water truly is the "nectar" of good health.

As a little added insurance, I take a multivitamin each day. It's not essential, but if my day's worth of well-planned meals "bites the dust" when unexpected events intrude on my regular routine, my body still gets its vital nutrients.

The calories listed in each group of choices are averages. Some choices within each group may be higher or lower, so it's important to select a variety of different foods instead of eating the same three or four all the time.

Use your Optional Calories (OC)! They are what I call "life's little extras." They make all the difference in how you enjoy your food and appreciate the variety available to you. Yes, we can get by without them, but do you really want to? Keep in mind that you should be using all your daily Weight Loss Choices first to ensure you are getting the basics of good nutrition. But I guarantee that Optional Calories will keep you from feeling deprived—and help you reach your weight-loss goals.

Are Healthy Exchanges Ingredients Really Healthy?

When I first created Healthy Exchanges, many people asked about sodium, about whether it was necessary to calculate the percentage of fat, saturated fat, and cholesterol in a healthy diet, and

about my use of processed foods in many recipes. I've researched these questions as I was developing my program, so you can feel confident about using the recipes and food plan.

Sodium

Most people consume more sodium than their bodies need. The American Heart Association and the American Diabetes Association recommend limiting daily sodium intake to no more than 3,000 milligrams per day. If your doctor suggests that you limit your sodium even more, then *you really must read food labels.*

Sodium is an essential nutrient and should not be completely eliminated. It helps to regulate blood volume and is needed for normal daily muscle and nerve functions. Most of us, however, have no trouble getting "all we need" and then some.

As with everything else, moderation is my approach. I rarely ever have salt in my list as an added ingredient. But if you're especially sodium sensitive, make the right choices for yourself—and save high-sodium foods such as sauerkraut for an occasional treat.

I use lots of spices to enhance flavors, so you won't notice the absence of salt. In the few cases where it is used, it's vital for the success of the recipe, so please don't omit it.

When I do include an ingredient high in sodium, I try to compensate by using low-sodium products in the remainder of the recipe. Many fat-free products are a little higher in sodium to make up for any loss of flavor that disappeared along with the fat. But when I take advantage of these fat-free, higher-sodium products, I stretch that ingredient within the recipe, lowering the amount of sodium per serving. A good example is my use of fat-free canned soups. While the suggested number of servings per can is two, I make sure my final creation serves at least four and sometimes six. So the soup's sodium has been "watered down" from one-third to one-half of the original amount.

Even if you don't have to watch your sodium intake for medical reasons, practicing moderation is another "healthy exchange" to make on your own journey to good health.

Fat Percentages

We've been told that 30 percent is the magic number—that we should limit fat intake to 30 percent or less of our total calories. It's good advice, and I try to have a weekly average of 15 to 25 percent myself. I believe any less than 15 percent is really just another restrictive diet that won't last. And more than 25 percent on a regular basis is too much of a good thing.

When I started listing fat grams along with calories in my recipes, I was tempted to include the percentage of calories from fat. After all, in the vast majority of my recipes, that percentage is well below 30 percent.

Figuring fat grams is easy enough. Each gram of fat equals 9 calories. Multiply fat grams by 9, then divide that number by the total calories to get the percentage of calories from fat.

So why don't I do it? After consulting four registered dietitians for advice, I decided to omit this information. They felt that it's too easy for people to become obsessed by that 30 percent figure, which is after all supposed to be a percentage of total calories over the course of a day or a week. We mustn't feel we can't include a healthy ingredient such as pecans or olives in one recipe just because, on its own, it derives more than 30 percent of its calories from fat.

An example of this would be a casserole made with 90 percent lean red meat. Most of us benefit from eating red meat in moderation, as it provides iron and niacin in our diets. If we *only* look at the percentage of calories from fat in a serving of this one dish, which might be as high as 40 to 45 percent, we might choose not to include this recipe in our weekly food plan.

The dietitians suggested that it's important to consider the total picture when making such decisions. As long as your overall food plan keeps fat calories to 30 percent, it's all right to enjoy an occasional dish that is somewhat higher in fat content. Healthy foods I include in **MODERATION** include 90 percent lean red meat, olives, and nuts. I don't eat these foods every day, and I know you don't either. But occasionally, in a good recipe, they make all the difference in the world between just getting by (deprivation) and truly enjoying your food.

Remember, the goal is eating in a healthy way so you can enjoy and live well the rest of your life.

I was so impressed that lean beef could be used instead of ground turkey. My husband doesn't eat anything with fins or feathers. And only eight ounces for most dishes—I could actually defend the cost of 91 percent lean! I tried several recipes and each time my husband gave a thumbs-up, even two!... You've brought more than tasty, healthy dishes into my kitchen—you've brought joy and confidence, too.

—G. A., CA

I have fought my weight since I was a little girl. I'm now 66 and retired and still trying to lose weight. My husband cooked up our supper from your recipes. It was delicious and very filling. I'm at the point where I hate to cook, but I could enjoy your recipes.

—D. S., WI

Saturated Fats and Cholesterol

You'll see that I don't provide calculations for saturated fats or cholesterol amounts in my recipes. It's for the simple and yet not so simple reason that accurate, up-to-date, brand-specific information can be difficult to obtain from food manufacturers, especially since the way in which they produce food keeps changing rapidly. But once more I've consulted with registered dietitians and other professionals, and found that because I use only a few products that are high in saturated fat, and use them in such limited quantities, my recipes are suitable for patients concerned about controlling or lowering cholesterol. You'll also find that whenever I do use one of these ingredients *in moderation*, everything else in the recipe, and in the meals my family and I enjoy, is low in fat.

Processed Foods

Some people have asked how "healthy" recipes can so often use "processed foods"—ready-made products like canned soups, prepared piecrusts, frozen potatoes, and frozen whipped topping. Well, I believe that such foods, used properly (that word *moderation* again) as part of a healthy lifestyle, have a place as ingredients in healthy recipes.

I'm not in favor of spraying everything we eat with chemicals, and I don't mean that all our foods should come out of packages. But I do think we should use the best available products to make cooking easier and foods taste better. I take advantage of good low-fat and low-sugar products, and my recipes are created for busy people like me who want to eat well and eat healthily. I don't expect people to visit out-of-the-way health-food stores or find time to cook beans from scratch—*because I don't.* There are lots of very good processed foods available in your local grocery store, and they can make it so much easier to enjoy the benefits of healthy eating.

I certainly don't recommend that everything you eat come from a can, box, or jar. I think the best of all possible worlds is to start with the basics: rice, poultry, fish, or beef, and raw vegetables—then throw in a can of reduced-sodium/97 percent fat-free soup (a processed food) and end up with an appetizing, easy-to-prepare healthy meal.

Most of us can't grow fresh food in the backyard, and many people don't even have a nearby farmers' market. But instead of saying, "Well, I can't get to the health-food store so why not eat that hot-fudge sundae?" you gotta play ball where your ball field is. I want to help you figure out ways to make living healthily **doable** *wherever you live,* or you're not going to stick with it.

I've checked with the American Dietetic Association, the American Diabetic Association, and with many registered dietitians, and I've been assured that sugar-free and fat-free processed products that use sugar and fat substitutes are safe when used in the intended way. This means a realistic serving, not one hundred cans of diet soda every day of the year! Even carrots can turn your skin orange if you eat far too many, but does anyone suggest we avoid eating carrots?

Of course, it is your privilege to disagree with me and to use whatever you choose when you prepare your food. I never want to be one of those "opinionated" people who think it's their God-given right to make personal decisions for others and insist that their way is the *only* way.

Besides, new research comes out every day that declares one food bad and another food good. Then a few days later, some new information emerges, saying that the opposite is true. When the facts are sifted from the fiction, the truth is probably somewhere in between. I know I feel confused when what was bad for me last year is good for me now, and vice versa.

Instead of listening to unreasonable sermons by naysayers who are nowhere around when it comes time to make a quick and healthy meal for your family, I've tried to incorporate the best processed foods I can find into my Healthy Exchanges recipes. I get stacks of mail from people who are thrilled to discover they can eat good-tasting food and who proudly use processed foods in the intended way. I think you will agree that my common-sense approach to healthy cooking is the right choice for many. Because these foods are convenient, tasty, and good substitutes for less-healthy products, people are willing to use them long-term.

So don't let anyone make you feel ashamed for including these products in your healthy lifestyle. Only you can decide what's best for you and your family's needs. Part of living a healthy lifestyle is making those decisions and *getting on with life.*

My husband has been a diabetic for forty years, and trying to get him to eat right has always been a challenge. But boy have you made a change. My husband loves the food and it doesn't take me half a day to prepare. You have made a wonderful change for the better in my husband's life. Keep up the marvelous work!

—B. E., IA

CREATING A DAILY MENU

Now that you've seen the kinds of quantities and choices you'll be making on a daily basis, here's a sample day's menu that features a variety of dishes I've created for you—many of these are dishes you won't expect to find on a low-fat diet. All of these tasty foods are favorites of mine and Cliff's—and the recipes for them are easy to make.

Here's one delicious day to whet your appetite:

Breakfast: Lemon Pancakes with Blueberry Sauce
with 1 cup skim milk

Lunch: Shrimp Caesar Salad
Frosted Orange Salad
Peach Melba Daiquiri

Dinner: French Onion Soup
Frisco Salad
Molded Relish Salad
Creamy Mashed Potatoes
with 2 teaspoons reduced-calorie margarine
Chicken Breasts with Raspberry Sauce
South Seas Chocolate Tarts

Snack #1: Paradise Yogurt

Snack #2: Wacky Spice Cake

You'll see that this entire day—everything you'll eat—is based on Healthy Exchanges recipes. Do I expect you to eat like this every day? Do you think that *I* eat like this every day? NO. And NO again.

But I want you to see the world of possibilities, to understand just how varied and satisfying your daily food intake can be. If I didn't show you this, it's likely you might say, "I'm so busy, I'll just select some items from the Exchange Lists—some plain broiled chicken, some canned carrots, a slice of diet bread—" STOP!

Please. That sounds just like a diet—and you aren't going to live that way anymore.

Of course you can have cereal and skim milk for breakfast, just as I do on many busy mornings. (But I make even the most rushed morning meal a treat, by adding a teaspoon of nuts and some fresh fruit to the bowl, for a breakfast sundae!) But as part of your new way of eating—your "nondiet"—make a promise to yourself to experiment a little with some new dishes. Besides being quick and easy to prepare, they are appealing to the eye and make an ordinary meal into an occasion.

Let's start with breakfast. (I'm using Sunday's menu for this practice session.) I've suggested **Lemon Pancakes with Blueberry Sauce** (page 288) for today. (My grandson Zach *loves* these!) The recipe, which serves 8, calls for fresh or frozen blueberries, Bisquick baking mix, eggs, yogurt, vanilla pudding. . . . Does that sound like deprivation? Not to me, either.

Each serving of this recipe equals 1 Bread, ¼ Skim Milk, ¼ Protein (limited), ¼ Fruit, and 18 Optional Calories. I mark off the exchanges on my Daily Planner so I can see what I've eaten and can plan the rest of the day. (I also take my multivitamin and drink my first two glasses of water. Check, check.)

But wait, there's more! (Sounds like a late-night television ad . . .) This breakfast also includes a glass of skim milk, so I mark off 1 Skim Milk serving on the planner.

Lunch today features some delicious recipes that will delight your taste buds and please your eye as well: Shrimp Caesar Salad, Frosted Orange Salad (which is probably the most scrumptious gelatin salad you will ever taste!), and a luscious drink that I almost called "nectar of the gods," Peach Melba Daiquiri.

Let's begin with **Shrimp Caesar Salad** (page 245). Each serving equals 3 Vegetable, 1¾ Protein, ¼ Bread, ¼ Slider, and 11 Optional Calories. My Daily Planner is filling up slowly, but so is my stomach!

The nutritional information at the end of each recipe makes it easy to keep track of what exchanges you've used, whether you're interested in counting Weight Loss Choices, Diabetic Exchanges, or calories, fiber, and fat grams.

The next dish is **Frosted Orange Salad** (page 241). A serving equals ¾ Fruit, ¼ Skim Milk, ¼ Slider, and 15 Optional Calories. So much wonderful flavor, for so few calories and almost no fat!

Healthy Exchanges Weight Loss Choices™ or Exchanges Daily Planner

Day: Breakfast

Skim Milk	¼	⅓	½	⅔	¾	1	¼	⅓	½	⅔	¾	1
Fat	¼	⅓	½	⅔	¾	1	¼	⅓	½	⅔	¾	1
Fruit	¼	⅓	½	⅔	¾	1	¼	⅓	½	⅔	¾	1
	¼	⅓	½	⅔	¾	1						
Vegetable	¼	⅓	½	⅔	¾	1	¼	⅓	½	⅔	¾	1
	¼	⅓	½	⅔	¾	1	¼	⅓	½	⅔	¾	1
Protein	¼	⅓	½	⅔	¾	1	¼	⅓	½	⅔	¾	1
	¼	⅓	½	⅔	¾	1	¼	⅓	½	⅔	¾	1
	¼	⅓	½	⅔	¾	1						
Bread	¼	⅓	½	⅔	¾	1	¼	⅓	½	⅔	¾	1
	¼	⅓	½	⅔	¾	1	¼	⅓	½	⅔	¾	1
	¼	⅓	½	⅔	¾	1						
Slider	¼	⅓	½	⅔	¾	1	¼	⅓	½	⅔	¾	1
	¼	⅓	½	⅔	¾	1	¼	⅓	½	⅔	¾	1

Optional Calories									
	10	20	30	40	50	60	70	80	90
	100	110	120	130	140	150	160	170	180

Water

Vitamin

Remember, if you require more or fewer selections because of your personal needs, adjust your daily intake accordingly. This chart is intended to be only a guide in helping you count your daily selections. After using your Skim Milk, Fruit, Protein, or Bread selections for the day, use additional choices for these in the Slider.

The topper for this Sunday lunch is **Peach Melba Daiquiri** (page 292). Each serving equals 1 Fruit and 10 Optional Calories.

Marking Your Exchanges

Remember, each bar on the Planner represents one exchange. You'll see it's marked off in quarters and in thirds. If you get confused, remember some basic math: *four* quarters in one bar, *three* thirds. If you've marked off a half, and need to mark off an additional third, you have a couple of ways to do so. Either start marking another bar in that exchange group, or remember that one half equals three-sixths, and one third equals two-sixths. So—you've used five-sixths of one exchange so far. Yes, but what about mixing quarters and thirds?

I've tried to keep the math simple here, and throughout this book I will keep reminding you that *very little in life works out perfectly*. But, okay, quarters and thirds can be measured together by changing into twelfths. A quarter is three-twelfths; a third is four-twelfths; a half is six-twelfths, two-thirds is eight-twelfths, and three-quarters is nine-twelfths. Wasn't that easy? Well, easier now than in the fourth grade learning fractions for the first time.

Two meals down, tummy full, and an afternoon on the sofa reading the paper. Well, yes, you *could*, but why not gather the family for a group walk to the park, or maybe share a bike ride around town? I've read that exercising moderately *after* a meal actually helps burn those calories more easily. I'm all for that! Don't forget to drink some water between meals—it's good, and good for you.

Let's look ahead to dinner, as well as two planned snacks. (This program will let me lose weight? Yes!) The menu calls for **French Onion Soup** (page 232), **Frisco Salad** (page 241), **Molded Relish Salad** (page 242), **Chicken Breasts with Raspberry Sauce** (page 256), **Creamy Mashed Potatoes** (page 251), and **South Seas Chocolate Tarts** (page 276). Today's snacks feature **Paradise Yogurt** (page 291) and **Wacky Spice Cake** (page 277).

Take them one at a time to write in your Planner.

French Onion Soup: 1½ Vegetable, ¾ Bread, ¼ Protein, 18 Optional Calories

Frisco Salad: 2½ Vegetable, ½ Protein (limited), ¼ Slider

Molded Relish Salad: ⅔ Vegetable, 4 Optional Calories
Chicken Breasts with Raspberry Sauce: 3 Protein, 1 Fruit, ¼ Fat
Creamy Mashed Potatoes: 1 Bread, ½ Skim Milk, 4 Optional Calories (plus 2 Fat for 2 teaspoons reduced-calorie margarine)
South Seas Chocolate Tarts: 1 Bread, ⅓ Fruit, ⅓ Skim Milk, ½ Slider, 11 Optional Calories
and your two snacks:
Paradise Yogurt: 1 Skim Milk
Wacky Spice Cake: 1 Bread, ½ Fruit, 6 Optional Calories

Will there be enough hours in the day to eat all that? You may wonder!

"Wait, I Don't Have Enough Exchanges!"

Now, as you're checking off these exchanges on your Planner, you may notice that —oh, no!—you've gone over the allotted number of exchanges. You're "supposed" to have two skim milks, but you have 3⅓. How can that be? You're supposed to eat 3 fruits, but this menu provides for more.

I'm glad you asked! The answer is your *Sliders.* Some people view Sliders as only for special treats like pie, and feel they shouldn't use them if they can "help it." As for your daily "bank" of Optional Calories, many people tell themselves that *not* using these "extra" calories will help them lose weight faster. Now, doesn't that sound like living with deprivation, surviving in diet mode? You can't live that way for a lifetime, and before you know it, you could be back making unhealthy choices and losing ground.

If the writing and the charting and the planning seem like too much work right now, don't despair. Trust me, it becomes easier very quickly. But I hope before much time passes—a month or two at most—you'll only be keeping your daily planner *one day a week.* Many programs ask you to keep a food diary every day, but I found that it was best for me to do it only one day out of seven. I think that writing it all down just once a week gets you out of the "diet" mode and into living healthily. That one day a week—which I call Reality Check Day—when you're accountable to yourself keeps you from backsliding, so you're always going forward.

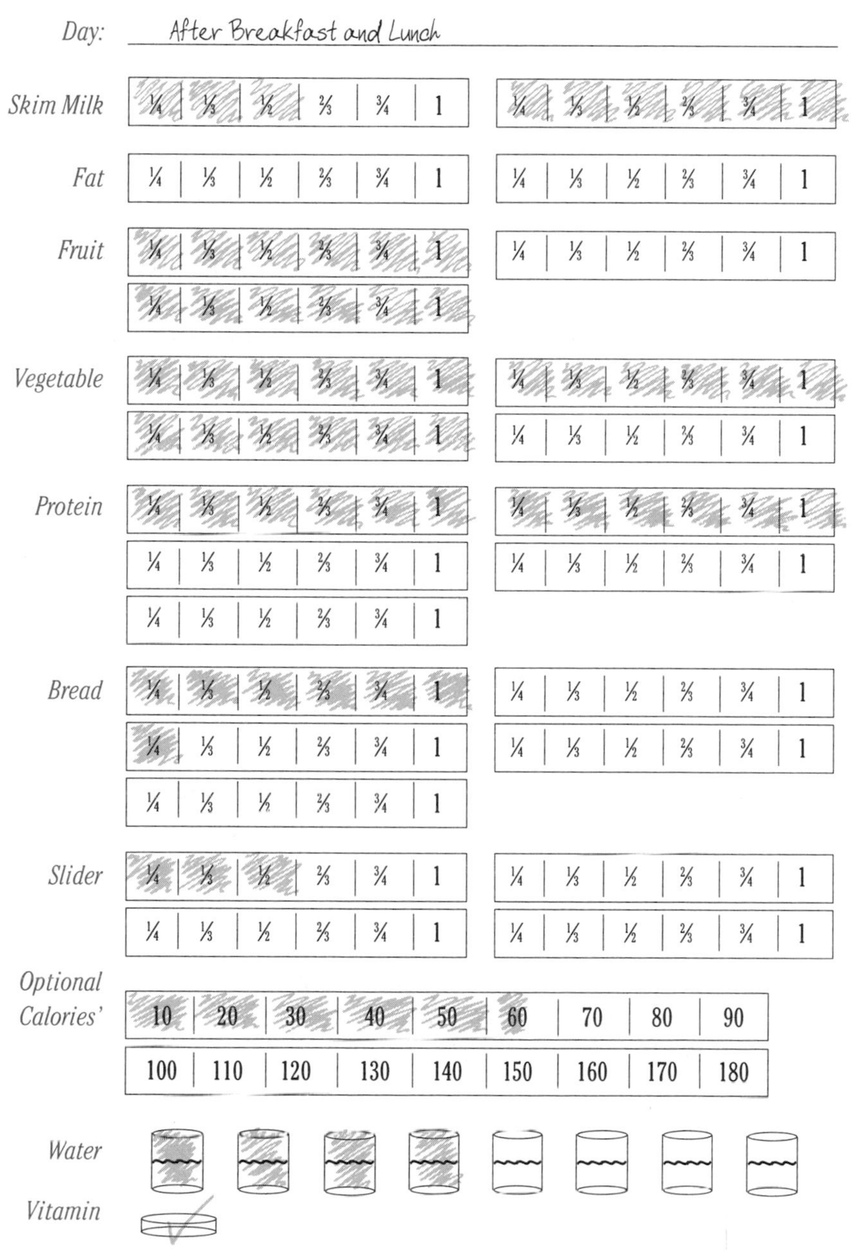

Healthy Exchanges Weight Loss Choices™
or Exchanges Daily Planner
Day: After Breakfast and Lunch
Skim Milk
Fat
Fruit
Vegetable
Protein
Bread
Slider
¼ ⅓ ½ ⅔ ¾ 1
Optional Calories'
10 20 30 40 50 60 70 80 90
100 110 120 130 140 150 160 170 180
Water
Vitamin

Remember, if you require more or fewer selections because of your personal needs, adjust your daily intake accordingly. This chart is intended to be only a guide in helping you count your daily selections. After using your Skim Milk, Fruit, Protein, or Bread selections for the day, use additional choices for these in the Slider.

Your recipes are great, really wonderful. My husband is such a big eater, but using your recipes, I don't need to feel like I have to stop him from enjoying his food, because they are so good for him. I can't begin to count how many times I've fixed your Healthy Jo's—they are the greatest thing next to sex, my husband says. Isn't he the cute one?

It's important to be honest with yourself. And if it helps you get started, you may want to write everything down more often than once weekly. But I hope that after a while you will feel so comfortable about what you're doing that you will graduate to the one day a week and stay there for the rest of your life. I still do it once each week—on Friday—so I can look back at the week, give myself credit for where I've been, and remind myself not to blow it over the weekend. I used to find that keeping a daily diary made me feel as if I were a hamster on a wheel, spinning and spinning and spinning, but not getting anywhere. I'll discuss this further in chapter 6, when I explain "Reality Check Day"—something I hope will be your very own Declaration of Independence from dieting!

As I mentioned earlier, you may choose not to create an entire day's menu from Healthy Exchanges recipes, and you certainly don't have to. But I hope seeing this will stimulate your own creativity as a cook, so that you'll feel free to adapt family recipes to fit your new healthy lifestyle. The ingredients are simple and easy to find, the portion sizes satisfying, and the possibilities almost limitless. For the first month, you will probably find that it involves some extra work and extra cost as you relearn your cooking techniques and restock your kitchen cupboards. But once that month is past, you'll be saving time and money cooking and eating the Healthy Exchanges way.

Now, I know that not everyone eats *every* meal at home. The Healthy Exchanges eating plan works beautifully for eating out, too. I've devoted an entire section (see chapter 8) to eating in restaurants, on vacation, and on special occasions.

Remember, though, eating is just one part of the HELP program. It's important to nourish yourself and feed your family well. But there's so much more to living a healthy life, and I've got a few suggestions to add a glow to your cheeks and a sparkle to your eye that don't come from gazing at a delicious twelve-foot-long buffet!

Healthy Exchanges Weight Loss Choices™ or Exchanges Daily Planner

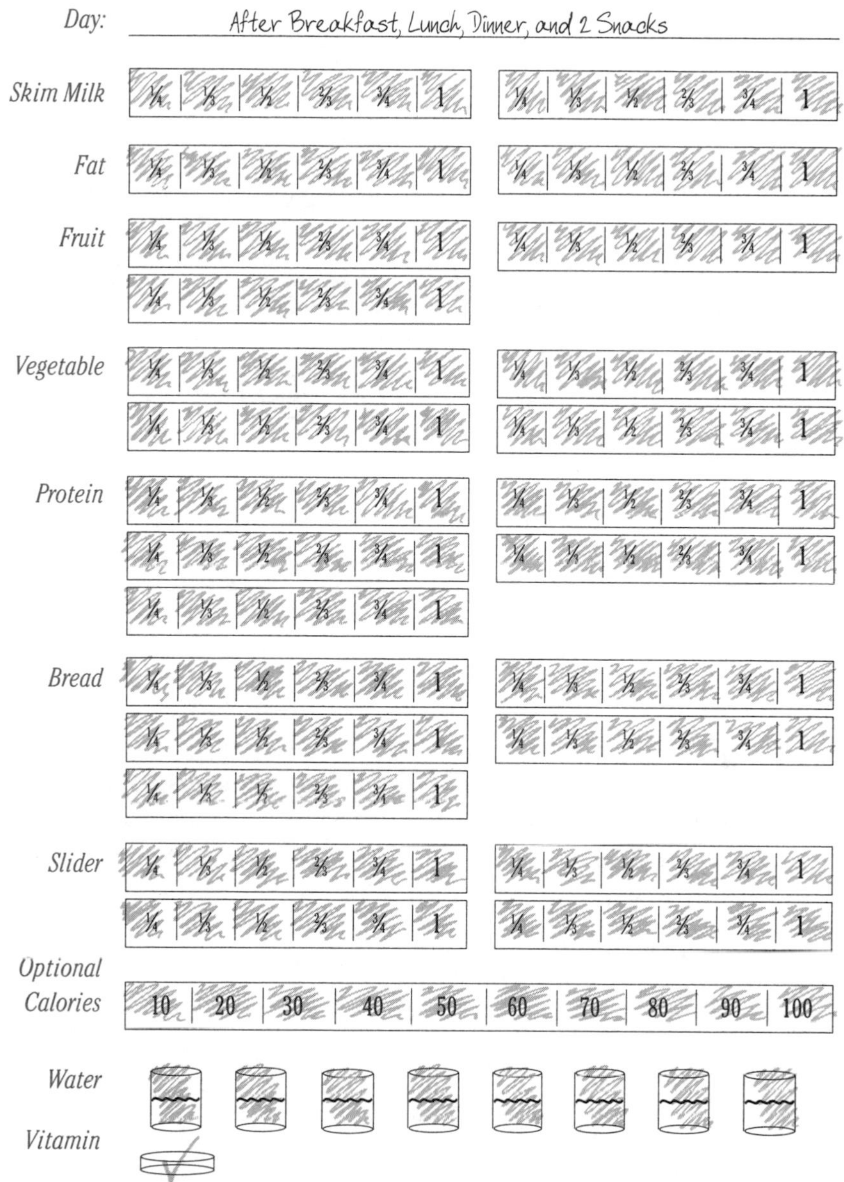

Remember, if you require more or fewer selections because of your personal needs, adjust your daily intake accordingly. This chart is intended to be only a guide in helping you count your daily selections. After using your Skim Milk, Fruit, Protein, or Bread selections for the day, use additional choices for these in the Slider.

Only "I" can change "fat" to "fit!"

—B. C., FL

Five

Making Exercise a Part of Your Life

If you believe that living healthily only means *eating* healthily, it's time for a change—a big one. I want you to take a fresh look at exercise—at how it can make you feel better, and feel better about yourself. Do you see exercise as

- A chore
- Hard work
- Discomfort
- An excuse for getting sweaty
- The first thing you eliminate when your schedule is crowded?

If your answer is "yes," then it's time to make exercise fun—and add a surprising amount of energy and enjoyment to your life.

If one of your HELP lifestyle goals is to lose weight, then incorporating regular, moderate exercise into your daily schedule can help you get those pounds off more quickly. And did you know that muscle helps burn fat *faster*? When you strengthen your body by exercising, just watch your increased metabolic rate speed up the weight-loss process.

Exercise is an important part of the HELP lifestyle—but it's vital to your long-term success to approach it with an open mind. For many overweight people, the word *exercise* brings back painful memories of being picked last in gym class, laughed at for being physically unfit, and feeling breathless and hopeless after the slightest physical exertion.

Did you know if you walk one mile in a swimming pool, it's the equivalent of walking three miles on land?

I know that feeling well—and I still remember what it was like when I began to take my first slow steps to better health. Making time for exercise, getting up early to walk, wasn't the hard part for me. Being patient about how long it took to feel physically better, to walk faster, was a little tougher. But from the very first day, I began feeling uplifted by my daily exercise effort. The walking became a calming thing, a necessary part of my life to keep my emotional balance.

I even used to walk around in the pool at our health club. The water puts up a lot of resistance, but it also takes a lot of the stress off your muscles. It was tremendously hard that first day to put on a swimsuit and get into the pool. *Tremendously hard*. But I kept telling myself I was doing it for my health, that I didn't care whether people might be laughing at me and how I looked in that swimsuit.

As it turned out, nobody laughed at how I looked. I think those fears keep a lot of people from doing what they should do. I can't promise that no one will give you a weird look or even whisper and giggle about your early efforts to get fit. And all those mirrors! But what's important is this: kindhearted people are not going to laugh; they're going to feel glad for you that you're doing something to help yourself. The few mean-spirited people who might snicker—well, that's their problem. When I felt nervous or embarrassed about some cruel people's reactions, I just reminded myself that their internal problem of nastiness was going to be harder to solve than my external problem of big hips!

I took it a day at a time. A lap of the track at a time. Ten minutes in the pool at a time. Sticking to it was what mattered to me, committing to a consistent program of moderate exercise would finally "HELP" me reach my goal of living healthily.

Never use a mechanical device when you can reasonably use body power instead! You can easily use up to 250 extra calories a day by adopting this attitude.

Some examples of this include: use the stairs instead of the elevator; ride your bike or walk instead of driving the car for short errands; put the electric can opener away and use the manual one instead; jump up to change the TV station instead of using the remote.

Finding Exercise You Enjoy

As the weeks went on, I discovered that what worked for me was making exercise *fun*—by turning it into a game, a challenge, with goals and rewards. When I'm trying to accomplish a particular thing, and I know that there's a reward at the end of the road, I feel renewed energy and a desire that can't be denied.

You'll be pleased to discover that you can start with little or no experience, and before long begin to develop your strength and stamina. I'll show you how important it is to establish and keep track of your personal fitness goals—and how easy it is using my Exercise Logs. Here's an example that may surprise you: If you walk for one hour at a brisk but not too strenuous pace of four miles per hour, you'll burn off between 400 and 500 calories, depending on your size and weight . . . and if you include a hill or two in your route, you'll burn even more! Do this every day, and even if you change nothing else in your life, you'll be burning close to 3,500 calories in a week—a loss of nearly one pound.

Would you rather ride your bike? If you can get those wheels turning so you're covering about twelve miles in an hour, you'll be burning 700 to 800 calories each time you ride—and burning off a pound in four to five days.

If lowering your cholesterol is your goal, exercise can really help. Numerous studies have shown that if you have a high cholesterol level, then change your eating habits *and* begin participating in moderate exercise and you'll reduce your cholesterol level faster than with dieting alone.

Regular exercise can lower your heart rate, improve your circulation, and make you sleep better at night. It even helps control your appetite and preserves muscle mass by using fat for energy. Best of all, it will just plain make you feel better, both physically and mentally. After I've jumped around in the pool for twenty minutes doing water aerobics, I'm so exhilarated that I feel I could conquer the world. How could anyone not like that feeling?

Enjoying What You Choose

Okay, so exercise can actually help you live longer *and* live better. Maybe you already knew that—and maybe you also remember how many exercise programs you started with good intentions and soon quit. Is there an exercise bike gathering dust in your laundry room, or are a couple of dumbbells lurking under the night table?

You're not alone. Many of us start with good intentions trying to do a workout we've seen on television, or one that a friend of a friend lost weight doing. Maybe you ordered an exercise video, but after one or two sessions, you were so sore that you stuffed it in the back of the videotape cabinet.

Let's improve the odds in your favor this time.

When I began looking for a way to add moderate exercise to my new healthy lifestyle, I looked for activities I could enjoy *right then* and still look forward to enjoying when I'm seventy, ninety, or a hundred and ten. I thought about what I enjoyed doing, and what I found fun. I chose walking, riding my bike, and water aerobics.

My first exercise choice is walking—in fact, I'm proud to be a "streetwalker." I walk the streets of DeWitt, Iowa, early in the morning—two to three miles, three to four days a week.

I much prefer to walk in the open air. I love to hear the early morning sounds and see the colors change and be part of nature. That's why I don't listen to a tape player or a radio. I want to be in tune with the bunny rabbits running across the road, I want to hear the birds chirping, I want to smell the flowers and the leaves. My walk isn't just physical exercise, either—it's a mental stress reliever, too.

Many people like to walk with friends, either because it helps get them out of the house or because their lives have become so busy it's the only time they have to visit and talk. Other people (me included) enjoy the blessed solitude of that hour just to think and feel and pray.

When I was losing my 130 pounds, I almost always chose to walk by myself, but these days, Cliff walks with me some of the time. Shortly after he quit long-haul trucking to work with me on Healthy Exchanges, he saw how much I liked getting my exercise this way, and so he decided to join me.

I walk a little slower to walk with him, but I enjoy the company. And, because he doesn't care to walk as far as I do, we usually walk together until he's ready to stop; we plan it so we're close to the house, and then I'll add another mile or so by myself.

Here's the point: I don't *force* him to walk faster or farther than

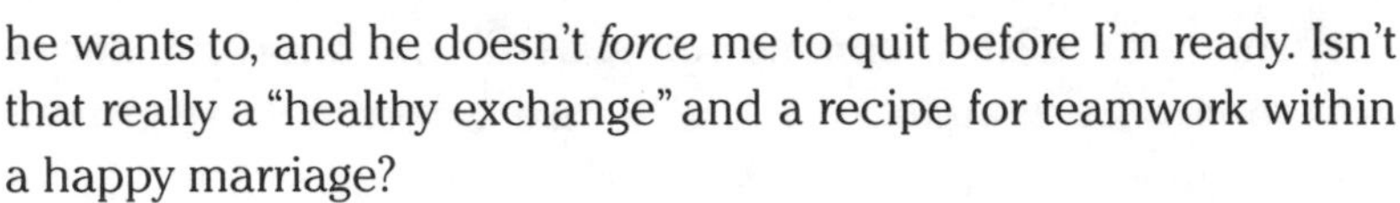

he wants to, and he doesn't *force* me to quit before I'm ready. Isn't that really a "healthy exchange" and a recipe for teamwork within a happy marriage?

Taking My Walk Indoors

When the weather's bad or cold, you'll also find me going up to the Hart Center (our local health club) and walking around the indoor track. If it's raining, or below freezing, or icy and snowy, then I prefer to walk up there.

Sometimes I don't have time to walk outside or at the health club. If I have an early radio or TV interview, or a deadline to meet, or I have to cook up a lot of food because I'm catering a speaking engagement, I walk my house.

You heard me right—I just walk around the family room, where we've had the Healthy Exchanges office for the past several years. I used to walk around the entire house, but when we got new carpeting, Cliff didn't want me to wear it out too quickly. I try to walk for twenty minutes at a time, which usually means I cover about a mile. I put the radio on, the peppiest music I can find, and I walk to the beat until I've covered the distance. If I manage to do it a couple of times during the morning, I know I'll have gotten in at least a couple of miles.

I did try out one of those treadmills that are so hot right now, but I never really got into using it. I don't have a place to keep it out all the time—few of us do—and I used to wake Cliff up moving it out of the bedroom into the family room to set it up.

I think it's a great piece of equipment for people who find it hard to get out—moms with young babies to care for, for example. But it just wasn't for me. Live and learn, I guess.

When we're on the road (which often seems to be *all* the time!), Cliff and I have learned to fit our walks in whenever and wherever we can. We've walked through malls in more than twenty states. I also walk the halls of our motel or hotel.

That might sound a little funny, but I've always been an early riser, and this way I can use the quiet time to get my walk in. I never know what might be safe outside in these unfamiliar towns, especially early in the morning, but this way *I do what I can.*

Then, when Cliff stops for gas, I "walk the car." I go around the gas pumps for however long it takes for him to fill up the gas tank. Maybe it's just five minutes of movement, but it's a good idea during a long drive to get up and move around. I won't do this when it's raining or in the harshest of winters, but I've found it's a good way to use the time that otherwise might slip away. Five minutes here and five minutes there quickly add up to a half hour of exercise you might not manage to fit in on a busy travel day. And all those drops of sweat will eventually fill the bucket of fitness right to the top!

Biking to Fitness

My bike is my car in town. Even in winter you'll see it parked out on the porch. Cliff gave up putting it away in the garage. Seemed that every time he tried to tell me that winter was finally here and I'd have to quit riding it, we'd have a good day and I'd pull it out and go pedaling off. Recently, he's begun teasing me that for Christmas he should give me a "heat houser" and snow tires for it. (For those of you who don't know what a heat houser is, it's something they put on farm tractors so they can ride them in all kinds of weather!)

I ride a mountain bike with three speeds and regular handlebars, so I can sit up straight—none of this crouching down so you can't see nature. If you haven't ridden since childhood, you may feel doubtful about climbing on again, but give it a try.

I did find the bike seat a little uncomfortable the first few times I rode. I also wondered what anyone watching me would think of the rear view.

Then I reminded myself that I was doing this for *me*, not for the approval of anyone watching. If it bothered them, I decided, let them turn their eyes away. Besides, the more I pedaled, the less rear view there was to gaze at.

Before long, I invested in a comfortable bike seat, one with sturdy springs. On any average day (except in the dead of winter), I easily put five miles on my bike just running errands in town. I'm lucky that here in DeWitt we don't have to worry about anyone stealing our bikes. I park mine outside the market, the post office,

even ride it down to our new office building. If your town is a little less secure, invest in a good lock, too, but keep riding! In fact, once you start, you'll probably wonder what took you so long!

People here have said they wouldn't recognize me if I wasn't riding my bike everywhere. Just think of me as the Jessica Fletcher of DeWitt, Iowa. Instead of searching out clues to the latest murder in Cabot Cove, I'm hot on the trail of new fat- and sugar-free products and lifelong good health!

The Water's Fine . . .

Another exercise I've found especially enjoyable is water aerobics. I don't usually go to a class—too hard to coordinate my busy life and the class times—so I just climb into the pool and jump around nonstop. I also get a chance to visit with anyone who happens to be around. I simply jump up and down in the water, and never even get my hair wet. (In fact, I leave my lipstick and earrings on, too!)

The water is a wonderful place to exercise, even if you never swim a single lap. I can do upper-arm raises against the resistance of the water, while keeping my head up. I also do leg kicks and stretches. There are dozens of different things you can do in the pool. I remember seeing one woman "milking a cow" in the water as an exercise for her arthritic hands!

After I work out in the pool, I sit in the whirlpool for five minutes, then the sauna for ten. It's part of my reward for doing something good for myself, and I feel so content and relaxed afterward. I like to lean back and imagine I'm lying on Waikiki Beach, with ocean breezes wafting over me. I walk out of there refreshed, take my shower and dress, and I'm ready to tackle the day.

The pool is also a really good place for people who can't do other kinds of exercises. If you use a cane or a walker, for example, you can move in the water in ways you can't outside. For people who think they can't do *any* kind of exercise, the therapeutic waters just may be their answer. Yes, it does take a bit more effort to work out in a pool, but once you do make the effort to locate a Y, health club, or public pool, you won't want to stop!

I don't do all of this every day, but sometimes in the summertime I'll ride my bike up to the Hart Center (about a mile and a half), go walk the streets of DeWitt to get in my two to three miles, then jump in the swimming pool for fifteen or twenty minutes. After taking my shower, I jump back on my bike and ride home. That's my ideal day, my best of best days. It doesn't happen often, but I enjoy it when it does!

That's *my* exercise story. Walking, biking, and water aerobics are my picks for the moderate exercise to keep my heart healthy and boost my energy. I chose them because I enjoy them, and because I'll keep doing them long-term. (You might also notice that there's nothing there that will get my hair wet. I decided a long time ago I wasn't going to fix my own hair, so the exercise I choose has to keep it dry!)

What Else Might Work for You?

Dancing. Exercise doesn't have to take place in a gym, or even require a minimum of sports equipment. What about physical exertion you don't think of as exercise because it's just plain fun? I love to dance—particularly ballroom dancing. Cliff doesn't enjoy it as much as I do, so I dance with my grandbabies. (Because they're so little, they're not embarrassed about it yet. I used to do it with my kids when they were little, dance around the kitchen table and sing along to the music.) Remember, before aerobics had an official name, people simply danced to their favorite songs and got their hearts pumping. Try it sometime—put on a good song and, even if you just move around for the three minutes the song plays, that's three more minutes of movement than you'd done before. If you're a dancer at heart, why not plan a regular evening out with friends who share your interest, or if you're really good, offer to teach a class at your local community center.

One of my older male subscribers wrote to tell me he liked to go square dancing. That's a really good exercise, and it's also a great way to get out of the house and spend time with friendly people. Another friend does country line dancing—it's as good for you as aerobics, and even more social because most groups include both men and women. If country music is your favorite, a regular date for kicking up your heels might be a great choice for you.

Did you know that exercise and water consumption have a direct correlation? Under normal circumstances, everyone needs eight to ten cups of water a day, but when you are doing regular exercise, you require more.

It's a good idea to drink one cup of water before you begin your workout, and then about one-half of a cup of water every fifteen minutes during your exercise. Then drink at least one cup more about thirty minutes after you have stopped.

Weights. A lot of people ask me about using weights or machines to build strength and lose weight. I did once buy some little free weights, some barbells, because I felt I needed some more upper-body strength. (Most women do, studies say. But for all they say, we manage just fine to carry those heavy bags of groceries and lift our wiggling toddlers into a shopping cart!) The Hart Center has a complete set of weight equipment, and so sometimes when I'm there and in the mood I'll use it, just for a change of pace. I like the idea of building a little more muscle to burn more calories, but I've never really gotten into it.

If you belong to a gym that has weight machines like Nautilus or Universal, ask if someone can teach you how to use them properly. I think it's easy to feel foolish or embarrassed because of a lack of knowledge—but we can conquer that.

What looks like fun to you? What do you wish you could do that you haven't ever done, or haven't tried in a long time? What sports do you enjoy watching others do and feel a twinge of envy that you're not participating right along with them?

Most people I've talked to seem to zero in on the big three—walking, bike riding, and swimming—because they're easy to do and they're available to you no matter where you live. That's not to say that you shouldn't choose Rollerblades or a rowing machine instead. The choice is yours, and the truer you are to doing what you really enjoy, the more likely it is that you'll stick with it.

Making Movement a Regular Part of Your Day

You've already seen some ways I manage to "squeeze" extra minutes of exercise into my busy schedule. I believe that everything we do adds up, and I've looked for ways to stretch my muscles, burn a few extra calories, and increase my feelings of health and well-being.

For instance, I climb the stairs in my house a few extra times a day. We have a basement down a long flight of stairs, so I decided to go up and down the stairs—on purpose—at least five times a day, plus another five just doing things that need doing every day. I try to do a version of this anywhere I go. No matter where I am, I use the stairs to come down. Motels, hotels, offices . . . If it's three to five flights or less, I will walk up, too. If it's more than that, well, common sense becomes part of the equation, and so I'll take the elevator instead.

I sound like a real convert, don't I? Many people have expressed curiosity and interest in learning how I changed from a sedentary person to one who looks forward to getting that blood flowing. It wasn't instantaneous but much quicker than you might imagine. When I began to change how I viewed exercise—exercise began to change how I viewed me!

I would *never* go back to how I felt before exercise became a regular part of my life. I have the onset of arthritis, and before I began incorporating moderate exercise and healthy food into my lifestyle, it would take me about five or ten minutes every morning walking on the sides of my feet before I could stand to put my feet flat to the floor. My hands used to hurt a lot, too.

I believe there's a direct correlation between the healthy foods I'm now eating and the moderate exercise I'm now doing, and how I feel each day. My feet don't hurt anymore. I just jump out of bed and keep going for the rest of the day. I'm often doing seminars and presentations three to five times a week, appearing at events where I have to stand on my feet for two to four hours at a time. I would not have been able to do that *before*. And it's rare if ever that my hands hurt me now.

What Do I Wear?

Before I started walking for my health, I invested immediately in a good pair of walking shoes. You need good padding to support your feet and legs, and you should ask the salesperson for a shoe that provides stability, too. Good walking shoes cost money, but it's an investment in your health that will pay off immediately. Not only that, but if you add up the cost per wearing (and you'll be wearing them every day) they'll cost you just pennies each time you put them on. You've probably got clothes in your closet that cost less to buy, but you've only worn them a few times.

Some people find it hard to get started because they can't decide what to wear, or they can't find special exercise clothes to fit them. Well, I'm not into exercise fashion or fancy leotards *at all.*

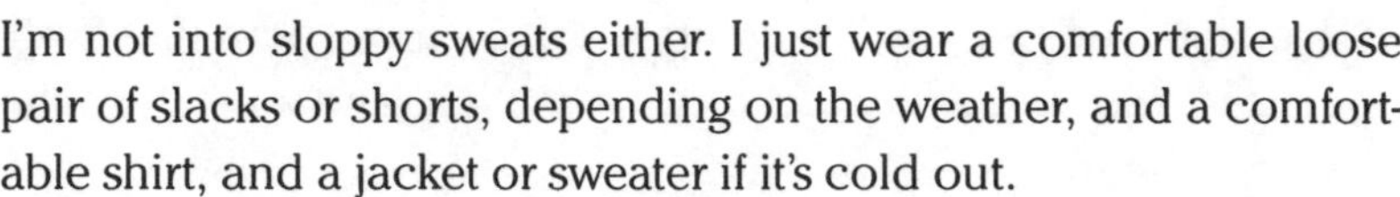

I'm not into sloppy sweats either. I just wear a comfortable loose pair of slacks or shorts, depending on the weather, and a comfortable shirt, and a jacket or sweater if it's cold out.

I don't even own any special exercise clothing—and I exercise just about every day. You don't have to wear a special outfit or a matching Lycra leotard and tights to get results from your fitness program. (If you choose to, great. But it's not necessary.)

I never worried about exercise clothing, but I did have a problem with the shoes. My feet always got so hot, no matter what brand of shoes I used, no matter what kind of socks I wore. But instead of letting that discourage me, I looked around for a solution . . . and I found one.

Now I only wear the Teva sandals—made like a running shoe on the bottom, but open like sandals on top. I bought them before they were popular, and I had to special-order them. I remember the day I first wore them and went to the Hart Center to try them out. Another walker saw them and said to me, "I'll give you a day!" It's now more than four years later, and while I do own a normal pair of walking shoes in case I have to walk outside in bad weather, I rarely ever use them.

I wonder if Teva would like me to be their poster child. If the world could see this formerly fat middle-aged lady in sports sandals, it might open a whole new market for them. Fitness and feeling good aren't just for young kids with great bodies!

Accepting Your Body

One of the positive side effects of exercising is coming to terms with your body, no matter what shape or size it is. Exercise can make you slimmer, it can make you stronger, and it *will* make you healthier, but it won't make you perfect.

When you look around, you'll see there are very few people with perfect bodies, anyway. (Okay, maybe on Rodeo Drive in Beverly Hills, everyone's skinny, but that's not the real world. That's Hollywood. The same goes for those models in magazines.)

Besides, you may look at someone and think he or she has a perfect body, but that person may not think so. It's time to stop worrying about what someone else may see. When you finally accept yourself, others will too. Your opinion is the one that matters most.

For me, it came down to choosing between self-rationalization and self-realization. What does that mean? *Self-rationalization* is saying, "I'm fifty, I'm big boned, and I'm hippy. I'm never going to wear a size 8, so bring on the donuts." Or the ice cream, or the fried chicken . . .

Does that sound familiar?

But *self-realization* is my choice. It's saying, "I'm fifty, I'm big boned, and I'm hippy. No matter what I do, I'm never going to wear a size 8. But that doesn't mean I have to eat out of control and wear size 28 either." Self-realization is about accepting your body for the way God created it, then doing the best you can—*the best you can*—and getting on with life.

When you change your philosophy to look at it that way, and you're doing the best you can, then it's of no importance what you're wearing or what size you are. When I was a professional dieter, I used to cut the tags out of things so no one would know what size I wore. Those numbers made me feel ashamed.

Then later, when I finally was able to buy a size 14 jacket, I deliberately hung it over the back of the chair so everyone could see I was wearing a size 14 at last.

Now it's more important to me that I just feel healthy, and I've stopped worrying about what size I wear.

People tend to use numbers to measure themselves instead of paying attention to how they feel and look. I think if the numbers are realistic, it can be fine to use them as a way to measure where you've *been* and where you are *now*. But if the numbers you're seeking on the scale are too low, or if you're reaching for an unrealistic clothing size, then you're living in diet mode—and that's dangerous.

Numbers tend to be the focus when people set short-term goals, not long-term ones. I want you to make the decision to live a healthy life *long-term*. Part of making that decision is deciding what's right for you, whether it's a clothing size, a destination on the scale, or an exercise program you'll look forward to every day.

I am determined to get fit and stay healthy and enjoy the rest of my life as a thinner person, and I need all the help I can get.

—F. S., SD

My basic program is simple: in good weather I hit the streets, and in bad weather I walk laps at my local fitness center. I can now do a mile in fifteen minutes, but when I began it took me forty to forty-five minutes of heavy breathing to cover the same distance—and I felt as if I was going to die! I never let myself forget that, and I give myself credit for how far I've come.

For ten months of the year, I ride my bike all over town. (You know I'd ride for all twelve months if I had my way—and if the Iowa winters weren't so snowy!) And three or four times a week I spend fifteen to twenty minutes in the pool doing water aerobics.

The key to getting the maximum benefit out of a fitness program, even a moderate one, is *consistency*. You have to participate in it regularly. Once you choose something you enjoy, you'll make time for it in your daily schedule, even start to look forward to it. If you don't enjoy what you choose, it'll soon become drudgery, too easy to "skip it just once" because you're too tired or don't feel like it today. It's a short way from skipping it "just once" to skipping it for weeks at a time.

Because Cliff and I spend lots of time on the road in our van traveling between speaking engagements and cooking demonstrations, it would be very easy for us to rationalize that we didn't have time for our daily exercise. But we enjoy and look forward to our daily exercise breaks. We use our mall walks to check out the bookstores to see if they carry my books. (If by chance they don't, Cliff usually manages to persuade them to give them a try.) Then we spend an hour together walking around. We do this *every* day of the trip. (And no, we don't shop as we go!) It's a great break from driving, and it energizes us for the rest of the journey.

Making Exercise into a Game

What else helps sustain my commitment to fitness?

I've found that if I make exercise into a game, it's much more interesting—and I get out there every day. Instead of just setting a general goal—like getting into better shape or walking a faster mile—I celebrate the journey by focusing on a *real* destination.

Here's how I've made my walking, bike riding, and water aerobics into a game for myself.

Every year, *on paper*, I walk to New York City.

Every year, *on paper*, I ride my bike to Los Angeles.

And every year I aim to spend a full forty-hour work week in the pool.

I do these activities in small amounts each day and keep a log of what I've accomplished. When I've walked or ridden my bike the number of miles needed and jumped around in the pool for the set number of hours, I celebrate with a nonfood reward. Instead of the cake donuts I used to reward myself with, I choose something that has a special meaning only to me—a plant, a wall plaque, costume jewelry, or some small article of clothing. Nothing too expensive, but not cheap, either. I want my "trophy" to last so that every time I look at it or wear it, I remember the occasion that allowed me to earn that reward!

I live in the middle of the United States, so New York and Los Angeles are just far enough away to be a challenge—and a reachable goal. Maybe you'd like to go to Florida in the winter, but you live in Minneapolis. Well, measure the distance, choose the beach with your name on it, and start putting in the mileage. You'll get there—on paper at least—and you'll be creating a better body for yourself by the time summer arrives.

I started by keeping a record of my workouts in a pocket calendar in my desk, and every morning I logged my miles. I noticed with satisfaction they were adding up, and I realized that if I kept going, day after day, week after week, I could make it to these faraway places. Making it a game increased the fun and gave me something specific to aim for.

You may want to set intermediate goals. Maybe Denver should be your destination, especially if you feel you want or need to reach your goal sooner. That's your choice. You decide where and how far you want to travel, and make your fitness journey to better health something special.

Start by keeping a Personal Exercise Goals Work Sheet and write down the goals that have meaning for you. Putting them on paper makes them more *real*, and more *reachable*. Here's the form I used:

Personal Exercise Goals Work Sheet

It is ______________________ miles from my front door to ____________________. If I walk ____________________ miles four or five times a week, I should be able to reach this destination by ____________________.

It is ______________________ miles from my front door to ____. If I ride my bike ______________________________ minutes a day three or four times a week, I should be able to reach this destination by ______________________________.

If I jump in the water for ____________________ minutes a day three or four times a week, I should have done water aerobics for ____________________ hours by ____________________.

Once I established my goals, I used a little notebook to keep track of my day's miles. Maybe you'd be more inspired by a chart on the wall, or by keeping a real diary of more than just the distance traveled. Some people find the time on the road good for all kinds of thinking and planning. If you haven't kept a diary since grade school, but you'd enjoy writing down your daily thoughts, do it!

What if you'd rather cover the distance by some other means? Maybe you'd rather use a rowing machine, a stationary bike, or a cross-country ski simulator. If you're truly adventurous, strap on a pair of in-line roller skates and hit the road! Whatever you choose, do make the effort to keep a log of your accomplishments—you'll be pleased to see how quickly the miles and minutes add up. You'll also see real changes in your body, your stamina, and your self-esteem.

Some people feel it helps to have a buddy to walk with or a friend to work out with. If knowing that you have a friend waiting for you at the end of the block helps you keep your commitment to exercise, then do it. I prefer that quiet, private time with nature. In a life full of busy days and work that involves lots of people contact, I find that's worth more to me.

I knew I was not going to be successful, until I decided to lose weight for myself. *Whatever I do, I keep in mind at all times that these dreams can be a reality within months, but it is all up to me! It is sobering, but I have gotten to the point that I know I can do it.*

—K. D., VA

A Day in the Life . . .

Everyone's schedule is different, as it should be. This will probably make most of you shudder, but I get up most days between 3:30 and 4:30 A.M. It's just when I automatically wake up, and I feel raring to go. I get up, say my prayers, and if I'm going to be walking at home that day, when it's nice and quiet, I like to do some thinking about how I want the day to go, what I plan to accomplish. Then I go to my computer and start working.

If it's a day when I'm going to walk outside, if the weather is beautiful, or if I've got enough time to go to the Hart Center and do what I want to do there, then I'll get up, say my prayers, and write until about 6:00 or 6:30. Then I'm ready to go do my exercise. I get home about 8:00 or 8:30, have my breakfast, and start my day in earnest.

Each day is different, but each day has some kind of structure to it. By 9 P.M., I'm done for—unless I'm out speaking somewhere. I

I'm down to goal but I've been there before, then gradually gained it back. It's important that we use every resource available to keep the weight off. I found that lack of variety causes us to "burn out," but perhaps it's not the program but lack of imagination. By having your tried and true recipes available to us, including those "sweet treats" that we enjoy on occasion, we can hold steady on the scales.

—F. J., IA

still get up early on the weekends, though I normally take Saturday and Sunday off from structured exercise. I like to say, *Whatever falls in, falls in*.

I might take a bike ride or a walk later on in the afternoon. I always cook on Sundays, which is still my number-one experimenting day, and before I prepare Sunday dinner, I often bike down to the grocery store. Sometimes I go for a weekend afternoon walk with family or friends, which is a wonderful way to share my healthy lifestyle with people I love. And when Monday morning comes, I'm ready to walk and bike and splash around, my commitment to fitness renewed.

Avoiding a Fitness Rut

Many people start an exercise program with high hopes and lots of energy, but after a while they lose focus, stop seeing their goals as clearly. The bike stands unused on the porch; the walking shoes spend most of their time riding in the car; and the commitment to live a healthier life slowly disappears.

How can you avoid falling into a fitness rut? Often, a special event can be just the boost you need to keep going day after day. After I'd been walking and exercising for a while, I decided to participate in a local walk/run. The runs had always been popular in town; my brother-in-law ran, and so did the kids. I used to sit on the sidelines, feeling envious and fully convinced those days were far past me. For me, the idea of entering a race or run was so remote, it didn't even seem like a possibility.

I was forty-six when I did my first race. For the rest of my life I'll remember the satisfaction of crossing the finish line. I was so emotional, so proud of myself and how far I had come—not just in terms of distance, but of changing how I lived my life. I saved all my race T-shirts (I still do!), and every year now I still walk as many as I can.

Walk, I said. I don't run, but I walk as fast as I can—and enter as many races as I can. We have a world-famous event, the Bix 7 Mile Road Race, that's held in Davenport, Iowa, every summer. It's very hilly and takes place in hot, humid August, but I look forward to it all year long. It's got thousands of runners and walkers, and I finish right in the middle of the pack. Each year I manage to shave a few minutes off my personal best time from the year before.

Another special goal I aim for each year is an event called "Ride the River." Every year on Father's Day, I ride my bike alongside my sister Mary for twenty-six miles on both sides of the Mississippi River. My sister and I look forward to doing it together every year, just as many families do. Cliff drives us down and cheers us on (since he doesn't like riding more than three or four miles at one time). When the ride is over, I feel tired but happy, and I almost wish we could do it again.

I could never have imagined doing either of these things a few years ago. Four years ago, I wouldn't have believed I'd ever be walking even a one-mile race or riding a bicycle around the block.

Now it's part of who I am.

The following pages include the fitness logs that I made up for myself. Feel free to photocopy these for your own use or just fill in a blank notebook. Keeping a log is like having a savings account book . . . just pennies a day deposited in that account soon add up!

Personal Walking Log

Walking Destination: ______________________________

Distance from Home: ______________________________

Week Of: ______________________________

Date	Distance Walked Today	Total Distance Walked This Week

Total Distance Walked This Year: ______________________________

Miles Left to Walk into Town: ______________________________

Personal Biking Log

Biking Destination: ______________________________

Distance from Home: ______________________________

Week Of: ______________________________

Date	Distance Biked Today	Total Distance Biked This Week

Total Distance Biked This Year: ______________________________

Miles Left to Ride into Town: ______________________________

Personal Water Aerobics Log

Water Aerobics Time Goal: ______________________________

Week Of: ______________________________

Date	Length of Exercise in Water Today	Total Time This Week

Total Length of Exercise in Water This Year: ______________________________

Number of Hours Left to Exercise in Water This Year: ______________________________

Personal Exercise Log

Exercise of Choice: ______________________________

Year-End Goal: ______________________________

Week Of: ______________________________

Date	Daily Measure*	Total Measure for the Week

Total Measure This Year: ______________________________

Measure Left to Reach Goal: ______________________________

* You put in whatever exercise you choose to do and decide how you want to measure it. Remember to make it fun and reward yourself when you reach your goal.

Think about your goals, not your limitations.

Six

Lifetime Changes—and Setting Goals

It's usually the destination that prompts you to embark on a journey, but the stops along the way provide a wonderful opportunity to measure your progress, celebrate your accomplishments, and reassess both where you're going and where you've been. Those stops, or goals, are the landmarks you pass. If the road doesn't have any, it can feel barren, lonely, and endlessly long.

Of course, it's important to select realistic and achievable goals, and to reward yourself as you reach those interim stops on the path to healthy living. Some of these goals are more easily measured than others: pounds lost, inches vanished, dress or pants sizes smaller, and love handles not so lovable anymore.

Others have nothing to do with numbers and everything to do with changing the way you live your life. Old habits can be hard to break, and new ones require constant vigilance to maintain. Maybe you've been telling yourself you're not ready to change yet; maybe you wish you didn't have to change.

Ready (or Not) to Change

No matter how unhappy or unhealthy we may feel, it's usually easier to stay where we are than to move forward, to move on. If we change nothing, we risk nothing—not disappointment over another diet failure, not frustration that we spent a lot of money on exercise equipment we used once and abandoned, and not discomfort over learning something new that might be hard work.

But no matter how we resist change, it is an undeniable part of our lives. Time passes, children grow up, and the seasons turn from winter to spring, summer to fall. For me, the Healthy Exchanges Lifetime Plan was born of a need to change, at a time when changing myself seemed not only possible but necessary.

I've always believed that love can be a powerful catalyst for change. Because I loved my children and didn't want them to suffer, I found the strength to change my life for the better, making a commitment to healthy eating and moderate exercise. Because I loved myself, I strengthened my resolve to live well for a lifetime by setting achievable goals—and by doing everything I could to keep a positive attitude.

But what should these goals be? How do we know what to aim for? There's a wonderful book by Barbara Sher with a title that says it all: *I Could Do Anything, If I Only Knew What It Was.* Once we figure out what our goals are, we have a much better chance of accomplishing them. Let's begin with a shared goal—to concentrate on the *L* in HELP—and discover why making lifetime changes will help you achieve better health and happiness.

Wait, you might be saying. *I know my goal.* I've always had the same goal—I need to lose fifty pounds! All right, that is *one* goal, a long-term one—but for now we're going to focus on selecting the goals that will help us reach the faraway, difficult ones. When the job is such a big one, how can you keep focused on the prize? So many times, I reminded myself that it would take months and months to lose my 130 pounds—and I'd feel defeated before I began. Remember the old Army slogan? "The difficult we do immediately; the impossible takes a little longer." Let's start there.

It's impossible to go from being exceptionally overweight to skinny in one week. Yet that's exactly what I was intent on trying to do when I allowed the "diet monkey" riding on my back to control my life. I wanted the pounds to melt off, preferably overnight, and I was willing to try any fad diet and weight-loss gimmick to try to

The harder I work, the luckier I get.

If you doubt you can accomplish something, then you can't accomplish it. You have to have confidence in your ability, and then be tough enough to follow through.

—Rosalynn Carter

make it happen. I refused to admit how long it had taken me to put on the weight I didn't want, but it was so much easier to wish the pounds away in a flash, easier than to contemplate what it would really take to lose the weight once and for all—and to keep it off by leading a healthy lifestyle from now on.

I had goals, all right: lose ten pounds by Friday, when it was already Tuesday (and even if I fasted for the next four days, I probably couldn't make it happen)! Or maybe I decided I had to lose fifty pounds in time for my birthday in three months, so I could fit into that size-12 party dress again.

The problem was, these goals were always unrealistic and unachievable. I'd become so overwhelmed by just thinking about the impossibility of accomplishing them that I would get discouraged—and inevitably give up.

How to Get Goals to Work for You

There *is* a way to make the goals you set work for you. First, make them realistic; then, be sure they're achievable; and finally, break them up into small increments.

What does it mean to have realistic and achievable goals? It took me a year to lose 100 pounds. It took me another year to lose the next 25 pounds. And it took another year to lose 5 more pounds. If it takes me another five years to lose another 5 to 10 pounds, that's okay—I'm not obsessed with losing more weight. But I am passionately interested in *maintaining* my weight loss. By taking the longer (but definitely more reliable) route of the HELP program, instead of the shortcut of dieting, I've cemented my weight loss and changed the way I live my life.

I know you had a reason that prompted you to pick up this book and start leading the HELP lifestyle. Did you want to lose weight after years of trying and failing at one diet after another? Are you desperate to lower your cholesterol to avoid dangerous future medical problems? Is it important to control your diabetes once and for all, to ensure your health? Or are you just seeking to *feel better?* (As if that weren't enough!)

Here's the good news: Those desires, those reasons, those concerns can be translated into realistic and measurable goals.

Then, once you've established a goal or goals, the next step is to figure out how you're going to monitor your progress. Jumping on the scale every hour on the hour is not monitoring progress; it's playing a game—one that *nobody* wins.

The key to success—what really works in achieving these realistic goals, and the best way to measure your progress toward them—is to break up each goal into small segments I call mini-goals. By deciding right from the start to break up your journey and take reasonable steps along the way, you'll be able to keep from feeling overwhelmed.

For me, losing 130 pounds was a huge, intimidating task to contemplate, but by giving myself a series of mini-goals—simply to lose five pounds a month—it didn't seem nearly as daunting. Instead of focusing on how far I had to go, I concentrated on my weight-loss goal *only one month* at a time—and kept myself moving forward as the pounds dropped off and the satisfaction of success grew.

Don't be afraid to give your best to what seemingly are small jobs. Every time you conquer one it makes you that much stronger. If you do the little jobs well, the big ones will tend to take care of themselves.

—Dale Carnegie

Setting Your Mini-Goals

Depending on the type and difficulty of your goal, I'd suggest a minimum of six steps or mini-goals along the way. By dividing your larger goal into these mini-goals, you actually make the big one easier to achieve. As you arrive at each goal, your resolve to complete the bigger task grows stronger, you've got a wonderful accomplishment to celebrate, and you've given yourself a moment to rest and reflect on a long journey. Best of all: Nothing breeds success like success!

I found that it's important to choose specific goals that have both a time frame and a measurable quantity of success. For example, I told myself, "I will lose five pounds in the next thirty days." Someone else might decide, "I will lower my cholesterol level at least twenty points in the next three months." Say the words out loud as you begin, and repeat them regularly—maybe each morning as you climb out of bed.

Think of these statements as affirmations: heartfelt promises to yourself to do *what you can* to reach these goals. Life is unpredictable and so is the human body, so it's possible you'll need more time to finish each task. *That's okay.* Another reason for set-

I reward myself for little deeds that grow into large feats.

ting these interim goals is to review how you're doing from time to time, and perhaps reset your priorities or make additional changes in your life. Maybe you'll find you need to allow more time for your exercise program; maybe you'll recognize that you've been less than accurate when counting your food exchanges. Maybe it's none of the above and you just need more time to accomplish your goal.

Reward Yourself

Everyone likes to get a pat on the back or a few cheers, something to acknowledge the distance traveled and the task achieved. But because reaching your HELP goals may be a private matter (unless you choose to share them with family or close friends), you'll need to take on the role of cheerleader yourself.

Whenever I reach one of my mini-goals, I applaud myself (I deserve it!). Then I present myself with a reward—a *nonfood* reward. I used to be good to myself with hot-fudge sundaes, but now I select something that will make me look good or feel good—a great-looking pair of earrings I've had my eye on, or a new dress. Instead of a plate of cake donuts to celebrate, how about a luxurious massage?

Giving yourself a small reward for reaching these mini-goals is a great motivator, too. When you have something to look forward to and a goal that you know you can reach, it helps you to stay focused on the bigger goal you've set.

I created the fill-in-the-blanks form that follows to write down my mini-goals. Spelling them out in black and white made them real—and harder to ignore on the days when I felt shaky or discouraged. This form is just for you to keep, kind of like a private diary of hopes and dreams. Or consider it this: a map of your future, *to be written by you.*

Add as many checkpoints as you need, and feel free to update and adjust your goals each time you reach one. This journey is a time to learn about yourself, and it's very possible your goals will change as you proceed on your way.

The Personal Lifestyle Goals Work Sheet

My ultimate goal is to ____

____

____.

I think it is reasonable to achieve this goal by ____________________

____.

Here are the checkpoints along the way I will use to measure my progress:

1. I will reach ______________________ by ______________________

and my reward will be ____

____.

2. I will reach ______________________ by ______________________

and my reward will be ____

____.

3. I will reach ______________________ by ______________________

and my reward will be ____

____.

4. I will reach ______________________ by ______________________

and my reward will be ____

____.

5. I will reach ______________________ by ______________________

and my reward will be ____

____.

6. I will reach ______________________ by ______________________

and my reward will be ____

____.

What should your checkpoints be? There are as many goals as there are people trying to make changes in their lives, and many different possibilities that have meaning. I've already mentioned some of the most familiar ones: to lose ten pounds, then another ten, to lower cholesterol by thirty points, or to stabilize your blood sugar.

An interim goal might be getting to the point where you no longer binge on food. Maybe you want to get in the habit of leaving food on your plate when you eat out, or to feel comfortable asking the waiter to wrap up half your meal to take home. Maybe your goal is to exercise three days a week, or to fit into a pair of pants. A goal can be as simple—and wonderful—as pulling up a zipper without having to struggle.

No one but you needs to know what your personal goals are. If there's something that reminds you in a positive way what you're striving for, then use it. I liked to hang a dress on the outside of my closet door, a dress that I was working to fit into. As soon as I reached a lower size, I would immediately purchase a new outfit one size smaller.

When I first started losing weight, I remember hanging a blue-and-white polka-dot dress on the door of my closet. I looked at it every day and imagined how I would feel when I finally could zip it up.

Well, by the time I thought I had lost enough weight to fit into it, it was *too big!* I wore it once, and then I took it in and wore it for a little longer. When I couldn't wear it anymore, I gave it away.

Even though the rule of thumb is for every ten pounds you lose, you go down a size, I've found that it's not really true. For me it was more like fifteen or twenty pounds between sizes. So don't get discouraged by a number on the scale; concentrate on how you feel and try to find clothing that makes you feel good. No one but you knows what size something is, but if you look and feel good in it, everyone will notice that.

Some goals are small but still very meaningful. I remember one man telling me how happy he was that he could finally bend over and tie his shoelaces, and he could reach around to scratch his back. I shared his joy at these accomplishments, because they reminded me that progress on the road to becoming healthy is measured in far more ways than any scale or tape can reveal.

Monitoring Your Progress—with Reality Check Day™

Did you ever start a diet on a Monday and, after being "good" at breakfast and lunch, feel compelled to check yourself in the mirror and jump on the scale by 4 P.M.? *You're not alone.* Wanting to see instant results, constantly looking to see "if it's working," is another symptom of "just dieting." You tell yourself you're looking for positive reinforcement, but often what you're really looking for, even expecting, is evidence that the diet's no good, that you're already failing, so why give it another minute . . . especially when there's a box of cookies with your name on it?

You're not going to do that anymore, okay?

To help you declare your "independence" from that old dieting trap, I suggest you monitor your progress *no more than once a week*. That's what works best for me. I still do it on what I call my Reality Check Day. Then, and only then, I look at the numbers on the scale and tape measure. For the rest of the week, I concentrate on living my life, not analyzing the flaws in myself or my diet.

I'm not denying that we're all motivated by success, but here's the thing: If you check more frequently, you probably won't see much progress, and you risk the danger of becoming discouraged and giving up. (If you can't handle the distraction, hide the scale!)

I do my Reality Check on the same day each week, and at approximately the same time of day. I wear the same or similar clothing and take my measurements at the same spots on my body to ensure accuracy and consistency. If losing weight is *your* goal, as it was for me, make the process more fun *and* more rewarding by measuring your success in two ways—first, at the scale, during your own private weigh-in, and second, by measuring what I call the weight-loss checkpoints: neck, chest, waist, hips, upper arms, upper thighs, and calves.

Why are these measurements important? Exercising regularly can replace fat with muscle, which actually weighs more. If your scale shows a frustrating gain, or seems to be stuck on a particular weight, make sure you also take a good look at your body measurements—you could be surprised at how much you've lost in inches and how your body is changing for the better.

(Don't forget, when adding up your inches lost, count both arms, and both legs!)

Giving Up Living in a "Diet Mode"

People ask me, "Do you weigh yourself every day?" Or, "Do you really write down everything you eat?" I proudly say, "No." To me, that's living in a diet mode. My sister Mary has never had a weight problem in her life (sometimes I wonder how we could have had the same parents!). She never weighs herself or her food. Instead, she does a *mental* Reality Check.

I can never graduate to that degree—most lifelong dieters probably can't—but by checking in on myself one day a week, the other six days I'm not living in a diet mode. On my Reality Check Day, I weigh myself, I take the tape measure to my vital stats, I weigh and measure my food, and I write down everything I eat—*only one day a week*. By doing all that one day a week, I keep three ounces of lean meat from growing into six ounces, and keep myself aware of what I consume in a normal day. If I forget what I'm doing, or I start to consume more or less, I've got something to compare it to, and it keeps me on track.

I am now living healthily with the help of this weekly check-in. When I first began, it took me a couple of months to get to the point of doing it this way. Some people might get there as quickly as a week or two. Still others may take six months before they can give up keeping that daily record without discomfort or concern. My goal is that soon everyone will be living this way.

This is a perfect case of "lightening up on yourself" so that your body will "lighten up" on you. Otherwise, it's too easy to remain obsessed about all this, to be focused on consuming exactly five Breads or five ounces of protein, so that all you do all day long is think of food.

I may never be able to live "normally" naturally—with no effort—but I can live normally with my weekly Reality Check.

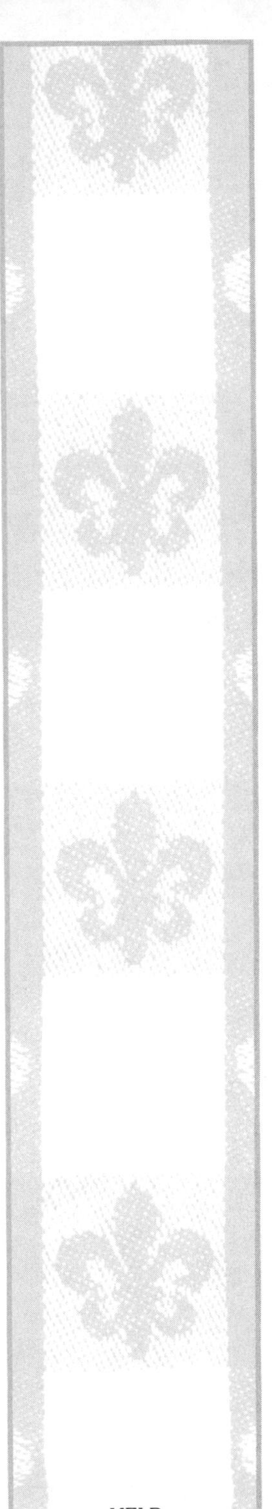

What If I Forget?

Now, I know that many long-term dieters may be afraid to do this, concerned that somehow they'll forget what they've eaten. Don't you think normal people forget from meal to meal what they consumed? You may fear that you'll go overboard if you fail to record every morsel of food.

But once you get in tune with your body, you'll find you just don't do that anymore. I get letters every week from people who can't thank me enough for "setting them free." They love the Reality Check Day concept, because it's one more step toward living healthily for the rest of their lives.

You'll know when you're ready, or just about there. It may take a few weeks to get the hang of it, but *you will.*

Keep your Reality Check Day charts private. No one else needs to see them. Put your sheets in a little binder that you can store in a private place. Then, when you think you're not getting anywhere, take a look-see at where you started and where you are now. You may be amazed at what you've accomplished.

All this sometimes reminds me of what it's like watching water boil. You stand over the stove and it never does. But when you walk away, those bubbles always seem to rise to the top at once!

Nothing is carved in stone, of course. If you're feeling a little out of control or going through a difficult time, if you feel you need the extra support, you may want to increase your Reality Check Days to twice a week for a short time. But as soon as possible, get back to once a week—and leave the old diet mode behind you for good.

Here's a sample form to show you how to fill in your own chart, plus one for you to use to record your progress.

Sample Reality Check Day (RCD)

	Starting RCD	Week 1	Week 2	Week 3	Week 4	Week 5	Week 6
Weight	210	206	204½	201	202	198½	196
Neck	15	15	14¾	14¾	14½	14½	14¼
Chest	48	48	47	46½	46¼	46	45½
Hips	48	48	48	47¼	46¾	46¾	46
Waist	42	41½	41¼	41	41	40½	40
Right Upper Arm × 2	15	15	14¾	14¾	14½	14½	14
Right Thigh × 2	26	25½	25½	25¼	25	25	24½
Right Calf × 2	17	17	16¾	16½	16½	16¼	16
Running Total Weight Lost	-	4	5½	9	8	11½	14
Running Total Body Inches Lost	-	1	4	6½	8½	9¾	14¼

Reality Check Day (RCD)

	Starting RCD	Week 1	Week 2	Week 3	Week 4	Week 5	Week 6
Weight							
Neck							
Chest							
Hips							
Waist							
Right Upper Arm × 2							
Right Thigh × 2							
Right Calf × 2							
Running Total Weight Lost							
Running Total Body Inches Lost							

Reality Check Day (RCD)

	Week 7	Week 8	Week 9	Week 10	Week 11	Week 12	3-Month RCD
Weight							
Neck							
Chest							
Hips							
Waist							
Right Upper Arm × 2							
Right Thigh × 2							
Right Calf × 2							
Running Total Weight Lost							
Running Total Body Inches Lost							

Making Changes in the Way You Live

I've lost almost forty pounds without feeling I've given up "normal" foods. I've been on many, many diets over the years. I believe this time I can do it, with the help of a good Weight Watchers group and your recipes. Thank you so much for sharing.

—S. H., IA

From the first page of this book, I told you that the HELP program was about making positive changes in your life. Often, we know we *ought* to change, to live healthier lives, but we find it difficult. Even if we aren't happy with the way things are, it feels like too much of a struggle to start doing things in a different way:

- Getting up earlier in order to exercise
- Shopping for different products at the grocery store
- Not eating and drinking everything we want at parties . . .

It would be *so much easier* if we didn't have to change.

I won't lie to you. Changing old habits for new ones takes real effort. It takes more than just the initial desire to feel and look better. Maybe you've tried to make these kinds of changes before, but after a while you found yourself gobbling cookies or shutting off the alarm instead of getting up and going to the gym.

That's the past. We've all got one, but we don't have to live there. When I decided to get healthy and stay that way, I told myself, "Don't let old failures dictate how you're going to live for the rest of your life."

Are You Ready to Change?

Do you live alone and think it's just not worth the bother and trouble to cook anymore, healthy or otherwise? I hear these words almost every time I speak to a group of people, and I receive letters every week that echo these sentiments.

Let's get one thing straight from the very beginning: *If you don't think you are worth the time and effort, no one else will either!*

If you've been thinking it's not "worth it," that it's a bother or too much trouble to cook anymore because you live alone, why don't you quit holding a one-person "pity party" and get on with a healthy lifestyle? Living healthy means eating healthy *every* day, whether you're dining alone or with others.

I think I know the "bother" and "trouble" of cooking for one person as well as anyone. I was a "married widow" at the time I decided to quit dieting and start living healthily. All three kids were gone, and Cliff, that truck-drivin' man of mine, was still a long-haul trucker. He left in his eighteen-wheeler every Sunday afternoon and didn't get home again until Friday night. It wasn't unusual for Cliff to be "on the road again" two or four weeks at a time. So if that way of living didn't give me experience in cooking for one person day in and day out, I don't know what would.

When I finally realized that eating healthy food every day was part of the well-balanced lifestyle I wanted for myself, I knew I had to make changes in my eating and cooking habits. Following my old habits—ordering two meals just for myself from the deli at our grocery store, stopping for a sack of day-old donuts from our local donut place/gas station, or driving each night to a fast-food restaurant to eat my fill of french fries and high-fat sandwiches—was no way to live.

Neither was going without food, or eating a can of cold green beans and a couple of slices of bread, or drinking some kind of diet concoction from a can because I didn't want to go to the trouble of cooking and doing dishes for only one person.

Jumping off that diet roller coaster and getting started on what became Healthy Exchanges meant finding a workable solution to this problem. I RSVP-ed that I wasn't coming to the pity party, and instead I went to the "bother" and "trouble" of making healthy food part of my lifestyle.

The Cooking "Marathon"

One solution I found right from the beginning was to prepare several meals at once. I cooked up a storm every Sunday while fixing our noontime dinner. In a two-hour cooking marathon I made a couple of main dishes, a soup, two or three salads, and a dessert or two. It really doesn't take much more effort to chop onions for two recipes than it does for one. And it's a lot easier doing dishes for several cooking projects at once than washing them all week long when preparing complete meals on a daily basis.

If Cliff was home, we enjoyed the fruits of my cooking marathon together. If he wasn't, I cooked anyway and enjoyed the healthy meal myself. (Either way, I consumed a realistic serving instead of having a pig-out just because the food was there.) After dinner, I packaged my own frozen TV meals for the coming week. I put foods that didn't freeze well into individual serving containers and stored them in the refrigerator. Then, during the week, I ate good-tasting food—food that was good *for* me, too.

In the mornings, as I rushed out the door to work, I just reached into the freezer and/or refrigerator and threw lunch into a brown paper bag. Because I didn't have to think about what I could find to eat that was healthy, I really began looking forward to my lunch break. When I arrived home after work, but before driving to my evening college classes, I quickly threw something already prepared into the microwave to "cook" while I took a few minutes to relax. I then enjoyed tasty food—a real dinner instead of a fast junk-food snack—before heading out the door again to school.

I was nourishing both my body *and* my brain. And the only kitchen duty I had all week long was the few minutes it took to heat up the prepared food, plus a minute or two to wash a couple of dishes.

I invested only a few hours a week in my cooking marathon in those first weeks, but the dividends of that small investment paid off big time! Because I was willing to change this one thing in my life, I was able to quit taking gout medicine, my triglycerides dropped to the low-normal range, I stopped popping aspirin to chase away hunger-induced headaches—and I lost 130 pounds in the process.

An unexpected bonus was all the free time I had during the week for other things besides cooking and eating—*all because I finally decided that I was worth the time and effort!*

A working couple in their late forties heard me speak at a couples' church group. Someone asked the usual question about cooking for one or two, and I explained how I had coped with food preparation when I was a married widow. Several months later I received a letter from them. They wrote that they now spend a couple of hours every Monday night preparing healthy food for the entire week. They told me that the freedom they reaped from not cooking during the week when arriving home tired from work is worth *every* minute spent in the kitchen Monday nights. The husband added that he doesn't miss a minute of Monday night football, either, because they have a small television in the kitchen.

Both look forward to their private time together chopping and stirring. *If a busy working married couple believe they are worth the time and effort, aren't you too?*

A single working woman in her thirties whose passion is sewing, not cooking, asked for advice about fitting my recipes into her busy lifestyle. I suggested she try setting aside time to make several meals in advance. She promised to try it and let me know. A couple of months later she called to say she couldn't thank me enough. She now prepares the "bare basics" for the week all at once, then just throws together a salad or quick dessert now and then, and has even more time for sewing than before. While cooking still isn't high on her list of fun things to do, she takes satisfaction in eating healthier and saving money by cooking the Healthy Exchanges way. *If a young single woman believes she is worth the time and effort, aren't you too?*

Another solution that worked well for me was sharing meals a couple times a week with a friend. We'd take turns doing kitchen duty and entertaining. Not only did we gain a night of freedom from the kitchen on our "night off," we also gained support from each other in sustaining our new healthy lifestyles. Occasionally we'd decide to have dinner together at a restaurant where we knew we could order healthy, tasty food and feel good about our choices.

An eighty-year-old woman told me that she and three other friends living in a high-rise apartment building for seniors take turns every week preparing a complete meal to share with the others. Sometimes they meet for lunch, other times for dinner. Each has to cook only once but enjoys four balanced meals with good fellowship during the week. She's earned quite a reputation for her Healthy Exchanges pies, she added with satisfaction. *If an eighty-year-old woman believes she's worth the time and effort, aren't you too?*

The choice is yours. It takes only a small investment of time and effort to prepare and eat healthy food, but the payoff—in raised self-esteem and better health—is greater than you can imagine!

A friend and I have been enjoying some of the desserts in the last two issues of your Healthy Exchanges News. *We make one of the new desserts, call the other one, and have our "dessert" at each other's homes. It has been great!*

—J. L., IA

Yes, but It Cost$ Too Much to Eat Healthy!

I can't tell you how many times I've heard that line. It's a good excuse to keep on doing what you've always done—and not choosing to make healthy lifestyle changes.

For many years, I repeated variations of it myself:

- It costs more money to buy leaner cuts of meat. . . .
- Lettuce and other fresh produce are usually too expensive. . . .
- I can't spend the money to attend support group meetings. . . .
- Health clubs are only for the wealthy. . . .
- And if I did go, think of all those fancy outfits I'd have to buy. . . .

How many of these excuses have you used yourself?

Yes, it does cost more to live healthily, but it can cost so much more *not* to live healthily, especially when you measure that cost in ill health and damaged self-esteem. Let's take a closer look at each of these excuses and learn why each one is really "penny wise and pound foolish."

It costs more money to buy leaner cuts of meat. It's no secret that a pound of extra-lean (90 to 95 percent lean) ground beef costs at least seventy-five cents a pound more than regular ground beef. But by the time that high-fat meat is browned in a pan, you're left with a small amount of meat and a panful of grease. When the extra-lean meat is browned, however, the amount of shrinkage is almost nil. At most, you'll get four real-world-size servings from a pound of cheap ground beef, while a pound of extra-lean will serve six or eight! So—the cost per serving is actually cheaper when you use the higher-priced meat. This makes sense to me, even if math was never my best subject in school.

Lettuce and other fresh produce are usually too expensive. If I had a penny for every time I picked up a head of lettuce or some juicy oranges and put them back down because I thought they were too expensive, my piggy bank would be overflowing! But even though I told myself I didn't have the money for fresh produce, by the time I reached the junk food aisle—and saw that my

If you really do put a small value on yourself, rest assured that the world will not raise your price.

—Anonymous

favorite treats were on sale—I'd throw twice as many packages into my cart.

Now that my priorities have changed, I know that my good health, aided by the vitamins and minerals my body gets from the fresh produce I eat, is worth more than the money I used to think I was saving by not buying it. Another unexpected plus: Once I began stocking my pantry with healthy staples, I began *saving money* on my grocery bill every week.

I can't spend the money to attend support group meetings. If you need the moral support that the reputable support groups provide, then you *must* find a way to attend. Many national groups, including TOPS, Overeaters Anonymous, and Weight Watchers, are well within the budgets of almost everyone. (TOPS and OA cost less than $10 per month to attend, while the monthly cost of Weight Watchers is under $50.)

Many people do just fine on their own, without the fellowship these organizations provide. But if you need the comradeship, guidance, and accountability, it's vital to budget for it.

Another option you might consider: calling a few friends to take turns holding your own free private support meetings. Keep the rules to a minimum and the enthusiasm to a maximum, and everyone will win at the losing game!

Health clubs are only for the wealthy. I agree that some health clubs are too expensive, and some members may act snobbish when you show up with a less-than-perfect body. But many clubs are affordable, and well worth the expense. Before you decide that a health club isn't possible for you, consider all your options: Have you checked the cost of joining your local Y? Will your employer offer to pay part of your membership through a company wellness program? (Healthy employees take fewer sick days and have lower medical bills!) Some high schools and colleges allow local residents to use their gyms and pools for a modest fee, or even free. And if all else fails, why not use your local mall as an all-weather walking track? It's free—as long as you don't succumb to any sales!

And if I did go, think of all those fancy outfits I'd have to buy. Who said you have to look like a movie star in order to work out at a health club? In the past four years, I've purchased three pairs of walking shoes at $50 each, plus a gym duffel bag for $30. That's less than $50 a year in expenses. I wear comfortable slacks or shorts with tops I already have in my closets. If anyone should be rude enough to comment on your attire, just smile and say that your self-esteem is so grounded in good health, you don't feel you have to try to impress others.

The Real Cost of Not Following a Healthy Lifestyle

Back when I was making up excuses at the drop of a donut, it cost me a lot more than I admitted to live overweight and unhealthy. I was spending $40 a month or more on junk food, $60 a month for gout medicine, and $10 a week on panty hose, because my excess weight strained and tore them after just one wearing!

Even more, I was playing Russian roulette with my health. If I hadn't made the decision to change my life by healthy eating and exercising, I know the future could have held expensive medical bills for all the diseases I was at risk of developing: arthritis, adult-onset diabetes, a heart condition, and more.

Harder to measure, but still costly, were the intangibles: shaky self-esteem, exhaustion, achy hands and feet, a feeling of hopelessness. The price I was paying to stay in my rut was too high.

Do you see what I mean when I say "It costs too much *not* to live healthily"? You can "bank" on it!

Invisible Goals

There are other goals that meant a lot to me, the kind of goals you usually don't share with other people. They may not be as obvious as the loss of 130 pounds, but they are just as meaningful and important as anything else I've attained.

For example: I'm finally able to get on an airplane and fasten the seat belt. For years, I was too embarrassed to tell the flight attendant that I needed an extension, so I would put my hand over the seat belt and put my jacket over my hand, so it would look as if it were hooked. Wasn't that stupid? I actually kept putting my life in jeopardy because of my size and my pride.

Here are some other less obvious but still noticeable differences about how I feel now:

- Being able to put a pair of panty hose on and have them last more than one wearing

- Not having my shoulders rubbed raw because of my bra straps digging into them from the weight of my body
- Not spending any more at the grocery store now than before, when I wasn't buying healthy food
- Judging myself on my actions now, rather than on my appearance

I won't deny it. I'm proud of my new appearance, too. One time I was walking downtown somewhere, and I saw this woman in a store window. I thought, now she's attractive—and then I realized that it was me. That was a great feeling! It wasn't one of the goals I ever wrote down in my book, but it was still one of the sweetest I've achieved.

My Anniversary Date—and Yours

One of the ways I've celebrated my accomplishments and focused the pride I felt on achieving new goals is marking an anniversary date of living healthily. Mine is January 4, and every year on that date, I set my new goals for the coming year. I think everyone can benefit from a day of personal reflection, to assess where you've come from in the past year and how much you've accomplished; and to look at where you want to be at this time next year. By writing your goals down, on next year's anniversary date you can do a real review.

One of my friends recently told me that she'd been following the Healthy Exchanges program for a full year; she'd only lost five or six pounds in those twelve months, but she was proudest of the fact that she kept at it, kept doing her best. If she'd gone to a traditional weight-loss support group, she said, she'd have been in and out of that program three or four times within that year. This time she wasn't looking for a quick fix, and when her anniversary date rolled around, she said she felt that was her major accomplishment.

We all know the day we start doing it, start living healthily. It's the day you know you are really not dieting anymore, you're just living healthily. *That is your "Living Healthily Anniversary."* It's a day that needs to be recognized by you and treated accordingly with rewards for every year that you are as well off or better off than you were the year before. (I'll tell you more about how I recognize my anniversary in the next chapter!)

Use this anniversary as a time to reflect on your life and your hopes. Ask yourself what you can and should accomplish in the coming year. You may even ask yourself if a dream you postponed is still possible, and what you might do to make it real.

Be honest with yourself, and remember that losing a *specific* number of pounds is not the kind of goal that you should focus on. Losing weight *can* be a meaningful goal, but don't fall into the trap of picking a particular number. If you lose fifty pounds, great. But don't make weight loss your *only* goal.

Here's another secret: Achieving goals is a great way to polish your self-image, and to solidify your pride in who you are and what you've accomplished. It's inextricably linked to the *P* in HELP, because nothing strengthens and sustains a positive attitude like reaching a goal you've set for yourself.

Lighten up on yourself, and your body will lighten up on you!

Seven

Building a Positive Attitude

Do you struggle with feelings of worthlessness, guilt, even hopelessness when you think about wanting to lose weight? Dieting can do that to you, because of the on-again, off-again cycle of success and failure it usually promotes. Sometimes we end up being our own worst enemies, doomed by negative self-talk and damaging putdowns that we rush to mutter before someone else does.

The fourth and final element of the HELP program is the pivotal one, the one that makes the other three parts possible. I want to show you just how important a positive attitude and self-acceptance can be in helping you achieve a healthy lifestyle and better self-esteem. By using my practical plan, you can quickly get into the habit of thinking positively about yourself. Positive people have the best chance of reaching their goals, no matter how far off and difficult those goals may seem.

I finally quit fooling myself into believing there was a quick fix to my lifelong weight problem. *There wasn't.* It took hard work and months of living healthily to lose those 130 pounds. And that was only a small part of the process. I depend on HELP every day to sustain what I've accomplished. And if there is any secret to long-term success in leading the HELP lifestyle, it's maintaining a positive attitude and accepting yourself.

So what if you're not a perfect size 10! What if you can't ever fit into men's slacks with a 32 waist? That's no way to measure our value as people. And yet body image obsesses many of us from childhood. It's a fact—no matter how hard we try, most of us will never have the "ideal figure" we've been led to believe we should struggle to achieve. Do many of your friends and family fit that ideal? I'll wager not very many.

Okay, so we weren't all put on this earth to look like movie stars—or to live like saints. It's time to accept ourselves as the unique people we were meant to be. Time to stop trying to fit into a "pigeonhole" of a size or shape that may just not be possible.

When I stopped dieting in January 1991, my body began to do with ease what it had struggled and failed to do for twenty-eight long years. I know what an accomplishment it was to lose 130 pounds, and that managing to keep it off for the five years since then is an even greater one. But I've still had to accept the frustrating truth that my bottom half will always be a size larger than my top half. It's a fact of life—and, short of surgery, I can't change it. But that doesn't mean I have to say, "Poor me!" shun all mirrors, wear only black, and eat everything in sight!

I chose to follow a healthy lifestyle because it makes me feel good, and I'll continue to do so. Eating healthily and exercising help me get my body into the best shape I can—and keep it there. I know that the longer I live healthy, the better my body will become—but my hips may always be size 14.

So what? At least they're a *healthy* size 14 instead of an unhealthy size 28!

The old song told us to "accentuate the positive," and I'm determined to do that in every way I can. I give myself credit for choosing healthy foods instead of high-fat snacks. I cheer myself on as I jump from my bed and go for my morning walks. And I celebrate every accomplishment and goal I achieve, because I've learned how powerful a positive attitude can be when you want nothing less than to change your life for the better.

Being Perfect Isn't Possible

As a "professional dieter," I used to say to myself, "I will be in complete control. Never, ever, ever will I eat chocolate or cake donuts again." And I would do fine . . . for a while. Then one day, I'd be paying for gas at the local gas station/convenience store and, before I knew what was happening, a candy bar or donut would jump right off the counter into my hands and be wolfed down in sixty seconds flat!

"You stupid fool," I'd say to myself, "if you can't even control what goes into your mouth, how can you control anything else in your life? You are nothing but a failure." After a day or two of bingeing and more damaging, negative self-talk, I'd say, "Okay, you got that out of your system. Now you can be perfect again." And I would be . . . until the next time the car needed gas.

Aren't you tired of being your own worst enemy? *I was*. So often, we set ourselves up for failure by demanding a level of human perfection that we wouldn't dream of expecting of someone else. Then we berate ourselves unmercifully for not achieving one impossible goal after another. It becomes a self-fulfilling prophecy: as our feelings of self-worth diminish over time, it becomes all too easy to fall into the trap of bingeing on hot-fudge sundaes or potato chips.

When I finally jumped off the diet roller coaster and started down the path to healthy living, I began to regain my self-respect. Following the Healthy Exchanges Lifetime Plan was my way of telling myself, "Quit playing games! Do your part, and your body will do its part."

I did, and it did. See how well the body listens when the mind makes a suggestion?

But before I got my body and mind to work together, I had to learn to forgive myself. I'm not St. JoAnna. Some days I don't eat what I should or even what I planned; other days I don't fit in my exercise—even though I know I'll feel better if I do. And plenty of times I fall back into bad habits or misplace my positive attitude. But when I do, I don't dwell on it. I forgive myself for not being perfect, and I get on with life—*doing the best I can*.

I'll say it again: doing the best I can . . . *the best I can*!

Trying to be perfect is dangerous, because the slightest little infraction makes you feel as if you've failed. You tried, you blew it, so

If you wait for perfect conditions, you'll never get anything done.

why not race headlong into a food binge the way you used to? We all fall off the health wagon sometimes, but by forgiving ourselves and climbing right back on, we don't lose the ground we've gained—or gain back the pounds we've lost!

Don't misunderstand me—I'm not offering easy absolution here. You can't just claim that you've had a stressful week, then gobble down high-fat desserts while pretending to follow your HELP lifestyle. But I am suggesting, as a weight-loss lecturer once told me, that you "prepare for war in times of peace." This might mean taking the time to prepare a low-fat/low-sugar healthy dessert, like my South Seas Chocolate Tarts, and planning to enjoy a piece as part of your daily menu. And if, by golly, you want another piece tomorrow, you can have it, enjoy it, and not sacrifice your self-respect to satisfy your hungry soul.

Use what talents you possess. The woods would be very silent if no birds sang there except those that sang best.

—Henry Van Dyke

Self-Acceptance at Last

There's an important difference between self-rationalization and self-acceptance. One lets you overeat and blame your genes or a bad day for not taking care of yourself. The other accepts your emotional need to enjoy delicious food but makes it part of a healthy way of life that includes regular exercise to burn off some of those dessert calories.

It starts with self-acceptance. When you lighten up on yourself, your body will lighten up on you. Mine did—130 pounds' worth! So try it. What have you got to lose but your excess fat, high cholesterol, and poor self-esteem? I know you're busy—I lead a busy lifestyle, too—and it's hard to make time to take care of yourself. But believe me when I tell you that you're worth it. And if you don't do it for yourself, no one else can.

One of the things that I believe sets Healthy Exchanges apart is my emphasis on finding ways to strengthen a positive attitude about yourself, to build your self-esteem. Other programs may talk about it, but they don't do very much with the idea.

It's more than just saying that you're worth the time and effort—a lot more than that. It's about forgiveness and moving on. Your positive attitude means knowing up front that you're *not* going to be perfect. So don't beat yourself up when you don't do what you think you're supposed to do. As long as you live positively most of the time, you're going to have more positive actions than negative ones, and you're going to end up on the plus side (not plus size!).

It's vital to look at all this long-term. When I was a professional dieter, I looked at everything as a short-term problem. I would never have said what I say now: "So what if it takes me six months to lose the last five pounds? Who cares?"

Positive thinking without positive action is nothing.

But I *do* care that I'm not *gaining* five pounds every six days. The time is going to pass anyway, whether you're living healthily or unhealthily. At the end of the six months, are you going to be healthier than you were when you began? Will you be breathing easier, feeling happier and more hopeful—or will you be depressed and down in the dumps again?

Most people with eating disorders are impatient. We want instant gratification. That's one of the reasons food is so appealing to us. We taste it with our eyes and start to salivate at its delicious aroma—and we want it NOW.

When I was getting ready to tour for the launch of my Healthy Exchanges cookbook, I wanted to lose ten pounds before I had to go on national television. If I had still been a prisoner of my diet mentality, I would have been fasting, or drinking diet shakes, willing to do anything in the short-term to drop that weight. But I don't do that anymore.

So—I didn't. I just kept doing what I do every day, and instead I lost two to three pounds following Healthy Exchanges. I let my body call the shots now, instead of chasing some artificial goal to please someone else. If the weight comes off, it comes off. (It'd be nice if it all fell off, wouldn't it?) If it doesn't, it doesn't. As long as I'm doing my part most of the time, I feel good about myself. You don't have to be a size 6 or 8 to be considered a success.

The Habit of Positive Thinking

Each day you do something positive, no matter how small, you are one day closer to forming healthier lifetime habits. And by taking the time to jot down your positive accomplishments each and every day, you can see how much progress you've made.

The fact is, most of us are pretty positive people, but we're just not used to seeing *ourselves* in that light. How many times each day do you do something that you don't have to do, but that makes someone feel better? When was the last time you complimented a neighbor on her appearance, helped an elderly person who was struggling with a heavy grocery bag, kissed a loved one on the cheek just for the heck of it, took the time to play with your child when you should have been mowing the lawn, turned off the TV and went for an evening walk, or made your spouse's favorite dessert (the healthy version, of course) without waiting for a special occasion?

I bet it was just a few hours ago, right?

And when was the last time you did something positive for yourself—got up early to soak in a bath while the rest of the family slept, or made a date to go bike riding with a friend because you knew having a partner would get you out of the house for sure?

Can't remember? I'm not surprised. So often we put ourselves last, praise others while ignoring what is right about who we are. I want to help you change that right now. Being good to yourself is one of the best ways to demonstrate self-acceptance.

It's easy not to notice these small acts or special moments in the midst of a busy life. But they matter, and so do you. What I suggest is this: For one week, keep track of them in a private journal. Give yourself credit for any action you've taken that makes you proud or happy. Maybe you made time in your hectic schedule to go for a short walk. Or perhaps twice this week you prepared a complete meal using all healthy recipes. If you handled a stressful situation without reaching for comfort foods to make it "all better," *write it down*! (I've included a sample form to show you what I mean and a simple form for you to use for this purpose.)

If you're like most of us, you'll be amazed at *all the things you did right!* After a few weeks of keeping this diary of your positive actions, I think you'll begin to see yourself in a different light. Because you've stopped focusing on failure, you've built the foundation for a solid habit of positive thinking that will support all your efforts to follow a healthy lifestyle from now on!

Sample Diary of Positive Actions Taken

Monday—Today I took this positive action:

I brought my healthy lunch to work.

Tuesday—Today I took this positive action:

Sandy and I took a walk together after dinner.

Wednesday—Today I took this positive action:

I prepared a casserole from the Healthy Exchanges cookbook.

Thursday—Today I took this positive action:

I got up an hour early and worked out to an exercise video.

Friday—Today I took this positive action:

Nothing much—but even though I was stressed out, I didn't eat junk.

Saturday—Today I took this positive action:

Ate healthily at a Chinese restaurant for dinner—no fried noodles!

Sunday—Today I took this positive action:

My sister and I prepared two healthy casseroles and three healthy desserts for the week!

South St. Paul Public Library
106 Third Avenue North
South St. Paul, MN 55075

Diary of Positive Actions Taken

Monday—Today I took this positive action:

____

Tuesday—Today I took this positive action:

____

Wednesday—Today I took this positive action:

____

Thursday—Today I took this positive action:

____

Friday—Today I took this positive action:

____

Saturday—Today I took this positive action:

____

Sunday—Today I took this positive action:

____

Finding Your Inspiration

In my booklet, ***Notes of Encouragement,*** I collected some of my thoughts—thoughts that sustained me, inspired me, and helped me move onward toward my goals. Here is one that sums up exactly what a positive attitude means to me:

> The greatest gift we can give ourselves is self-respect. Love yourself for what you are, and for what you are becoming through a healthy lifestyle. Pat yourself on the back when you lose a few unhealthy pounds. Rejoice when you make time for that walk in your busy schedule. Give yourself a hand when you lower your cholesterol or blood sugar count into a healthy range. But don't lose sight of your true goal of living healthily by reaching for the wrong goal of trying to obtain impossible human perfection.
>
> Accept yourself for the person God intended you to be. Get on with life. It's too short to do it any other way.

Never underestimate the power of inspirational phrases, whether you've copied down what someone else said or voiced your own deepest beliefs about who you are and what you aspire to be. Maybe the affirmations of your Positive Action Diary will feed the flame that burns within you, the desire to change your life forever.

I draw a great deal of strength and inspiration from my faith in God. My daily prayer is a constant one:

"Please, God, help me to help myself, *just for today*."

I firmly believe that prayers without action are doomed to failure; I also believe that actions without prayers are not going to last long-term. But prayers and action combined have the greatest hope of success.

I ask for the help of God, and Jesus, and the Holy Spirit when I pray, and together with the actions I undertake to help myself, I've found a recipe for success that works for me. Whatever your personal beliefs are, draw on your spiritual side to create the vision of the person you want to be.

I also draw inspiration from my own accomplishments. My Positive Action Diary still reminds me of what I've achieved each week, but I wanted a more visible reminder that would be with me always. That's why I have so many rings on my hands.

I wear five different rings (none of them very expensive, but

The roots of true achievement lie in the will to become the best that you can become.

—Harold Taylor

they mean *a lot to me!*). On my right pinkie, I have a sapphire-and-diamond ring that I got when I had lost 100 pounds. That was back in 1992. Then on my left middle finger, I wear a garnet ring to signify my loss of 125 pounds and mark the day I left my full-time job to devote myself to Healthy Exchanges. On my left ring finger next to my wedding band I have a pearl that I got on my two-year anniversary of living healthily, in 1993. On my left pinkie I have an aquamarine for three years of living healthily (1994), and on my right ring finger a black onyx ring for four years (1995). In January 1996, when I celebrated five years of living healthily, I rewarded myself with a diamond.

Thank you for your willingness to share these recipes and for persevering to find the answer to your health/weight problem. You just might have saved many *lives—not* just *your own!*

—J. G., IA

Anytime I'm even remotely thinking negative thoughts, all I have to do is look down at my hands and say, "Good job, JoAnna." I don't want to blow it, and *I don't want to have to take those rings off.* And so every year on my Living Healthily Anniversary (January 4), if I weigh the same or less than I did the year before, I reward myself with a ring. I'm going to do that for the rest of my life.

Yes, I may run out of fingers (so I'll just have to rotate the rings in order to wear them all, or start wearing two on each finger!) but I'll cross that bridge when I come to it. These gifts to myself provide an immediate and concrete reminder of how far I've come, and how much it means to me. There's no better motivation for living the HELP lifestyle.

Helping Others Helps Me, Too

I also draw inspiration from the people who write to me, my Healthy Exchanges "family members." I get mail every single day from people who tell me what a difference I've made in their lives, whether they've lost weight, or lowered their cholesterol, or stabilized their blood sugar. Sometimes they thank me on behalf of one of their loved ones who's been helped by Healthy Exchanges.

By thanking me for helping them, they are helping me to reinforce my belief that what I am doing really matters. Their letters tell me that Healthy Exchanges and the HELP program are not just something I did for myself but something that is actually helping others. Their support, the piles of correspondence, has helped me stay strong and committed to my healthy way of life. I don't look at those letters with vanity but with a kind of humble pride that I've been able to share what I've learned with so many other people.

While I'm helping myself, I'm helping others, and helping others helps me. It's a never-ending circle of positive energy, flowing between them and me, and I'm grateful for it.

You, too, can find a way to share the positive energy of your HELP program with others. Invite a friend to partake of a healthy casserole with you, and then take a walk after dinner. Your example of living healthily may be just the push your friend needs to make changes for the better in her own life.

I feel like a new woman. I am loving cooking again and my family is enjoying my cooking.

—S. Q., VA

Getting Your Family to Help

I started Healthy Exchanges at a time when Cliff was often on the road for weeks and my kids were away in the Persian Gulf. Being alone made some things easier, but it also meant I had limited day-to-day support for my new healthy way of life. I wanted to share what I was doing with the people closest to me.

When my family and friends understood what I was trying to accomplish, they gave me lots of support and encouragement. With Healthy Exchanges, I'd found a solution that worked for me, and they grasped wholeheartedly what I was trying to do. They'd seen me fail at one diet solution after another, and they were as negative as could be about those.

But now they know without asking that I'm going to be serving Healthy Exchanges recipes. And if they stop by around the time of day when I'm going to take my walk, they know they're welcome to come along with me. There's been no resistance, just acceptance that this is the way things are now. Of course, part of why it works is because they realize I'm taking care of myself, and taking care of them at the same time.

Cliff has had his life completely turned upside down, completely changed by my weight loss and the business of Healthy Exchanges. When I introduce him at speaking engagements, I always say he's "my truck-drivin' man" who quit long-haul trucking to truck me around instead. I like to add that he's just changed his cargo from farmers' grain and Alcoa Aluminum to a blond "dynamo"! It takes a strong guy to leave a macho profession like long-haul truck driving to work full-time with his wife in her business, and have the business be healthy recipes. Cliff manages to handle all of it with a sense of humor, even being addressed as Mr. JoAnna Lund (of course, Lund *is* my married name . . .).

Cliff's lost about thirty pounds just coming along for the ride and eating foods that four years ago he'd have sworn he'd never have agreed to taste. I still haven't gotten him to eat broccoli or shrimp, but he's come an awful long way with a lot of other healthy foods.

Part of me wanted my kids to know how they inspired me to pursue my healthy lifestyle from the very beginning. But when I first started with Healthy Exchanges, I didn't mention it in my letters to them overseas or tell them what I was doing the few times I got to speak to them on the phone. I figured they would think that by the time they got a letter from me telling them I had lost twenty, thirty, even fifty pounds, they'd be sure it was old news, and that I'd already gained it back, plus. What could they do, say "Good job, Mom" and make me feel bad if I'd already put it back on? I decided they had enough stress in their lives at that point, and so I decided not to tell them anything. By the time they came home, though, I'd lost about sixty pounds, and they couldn't believe their eyes.

My son Tommy, who just graduated from college a few months ago, decided during his senior year that it was time he got serious about living healthily. Forsaking dorm food, he took my cookbook back to school with him at semester break, saying he was going to start cooking out of it. (He was used to the traditional college diet of pizza and beer, so it was quite a change.) Tommy's been a real inspiration for some of my tastiest, most family-friendly recipes, and I plan to help him set up a Healthy Exchanges kitchen when he settles into his career and own apartment.

Becky Anne was always concerned about eating healthily, so our mother-daughter relationship has just been strengthened by my commitment to living healthily. Both she and her husband use my recipes. Her husband, John, does most of the cooking, actually, and he's told me that my desserts are dynamite. (From him, that's high praise!) He told me he wouldn't hesitate to serve them to anyone who came to their house, which meant a lot to me. When your kids serve your healthy recipes to company, you must be doing something right!

Pam, my daughter-in-law, now prepares my recipes on a regular basis for my son James and my two grandbabies. I think James was the hardest sell of all. He'd seen me lose weight and gain it back so many times. But he happened to be here one Saturday when I was feeling really lonely for my mom. That loneliness translated to a hunger for her Cherry Kolaches, her special pastry dessert. One of my fondest childhood memories was helping my mother and my grandmother make kolaches, and I just knew there had to be a way to make healthy ones. So I took all that emotion, went to the kitchen, and finally came up with a recipe I thought worked (see page 270).

James tried one but didn't tell me what he thought of it. But the next morning he was back before breakfast, asking for another Cherry Kolache. He gave me the highest compliment anyone could when he said, "You know, Mom, these are almost as good as Grandma's." I'll never forget that, and Pam now makes them all the time for James and the boys. It means a lot that my positive approach to solving my problems and living healthily has just become a part of all our lives.

Family support makes so much possible, and I think you can create a positive atmosphere at home by meeting your loved ones halfway. By preparing food with the flavors, tastes, and textures they've always enjoyed, you'll make it easy for them to meet *you* halfway and give "healthy food" a chance.

I know that when my grandbabies Zach and Josh stay overnight, it makes me feel good all over when they smack their lips in delight over Grandma's food. Zach particularly loves my Lemon Pancakes with Blueberry Sauce (see page 288). (I think your kids and grandkids will, too.)

Something as simple—and yet as remarkable—as making healthy desserts part of your family meals creates a positive environment for everyone to enjoy eating together. Instead of watching enviously and feeling deprived while others enjoy rich-tasting treats, those family members who are watching their weight or concerned about cholesterol or diabetes are free to share in the pleasure of the *entire* meal. I've had so many people tell me that they never ate so many desserts in their lives and felt so good about it until they met me! They always say this with a satisfied

You have brought back the enjoyment of cooking simple and healthy meals that my "meat 'n' potatoes" husband and I enjoy immensely.

—K. S., IA

smile that lets me know I may have played a small part in keeping families closer together. (Do you think they give the Nobel Peace Prize for creating healthy desserts?)

Triumph is the extra "umph" added to the word "try."

Making Your Dreams a Reality

For most dieters, food has become the enemy and exercise an unhappy reminder of gym classes where the overweight were humiliated and turned off to the idea of physical exertion. I created the HELP program to empower myself first, and then others, so that we could enjoy the foods that nourish our bodies, so that we could keep our hearts healthy with moderate exercise, and so that we could achieve goals that would build self-esteem. As the saying goes, I was sick and tired of feeling sick and tired from a lifelong struggle to lose weight on fad diets. Healthy Exchanges eating got me started; but the exercise, life goals, and positive attitude were the tools that helped me make a lifetime commitment to healthy living.

I think you'll discover that strengthening and supporting yourself with a positive attitude will spill over into every aspect of your life. When you approach a challenge with a sense that you can succeed at what you try, you're already halfway there. I am continually surprised and pleased when something I believe in with all my heart prevails against tough odds. I remember when we began planning in fall 1992 for a summer 1993 Healthy Exchanges Potluck Reunion, an event where we welcomed members of the Healthy Exchanges family from as far away as California to join us for a party to celebrate our shared healthy lifestyle. All they needed to bring was a covered dish to share, a lawn chair to sit on, and a smile; we promised to provide the rest, including perfect weather.

How was I to know that in the spring and summer of 1993, eastern Iowa and western Illinois would be fighting a raging battle with the mighty Mississippi River, and that they'd be calling it the Great Flood of '93! The site we chose for the reunion picnic was a beautiful park on the banks of the Wapsipinican River, a tributary of the Mississippi. Well, every weekend *before* (and every weekend *after*, as it turned out) our Healthy Exchanges event, it rained and the river flooded its banks, so we wouldn't have been able to hold the picnic. But the day of our party the sky was clear, the river was down, and even the ants were out of town. More than seven hundred people showed up, and we picnicked and visited all afternoon long.

Will you believe me if I tell you that the combined energy and positive attitude of those Healthy Exchanges "family" members made the difference in the weather? Okay, I have no proof, I admit it—but don't you think it's possible all those good feelings kept the rain away?

Every day of your life offers another chance to reinforce the healthy habits that you've decided are important to you. Being aware of each of these opportunities, paying attention to the choices you make, and patting yourself on the back for your accomplishments will help you sustain your commitment and renew your motivation. Keep following the HELP lifestyle and doing the best you can . . . *the best you can* . . . even if nobody notices. Then, one day, someone will ask how you stay motivated, and you can reply, "I've got HELP!"

You've got a wonderful journey ahead of you, one that will help you discover and reach for the many possibilities your life may hold. But before you head for the recipes and menus in part 3, I want to add some special support to the HELP program. In the next three chapters, you'll learn how to enjoy eating out and on special occasions, how to handle plateaus (yes, there will probably be some), and what I learned from all this about letting go—and moving on.

Part Three

Trying Times Are Times for Trying

There are no shortcuts to anyplace worth going.

Eight

Dining Out, Traveling Healthily, and Handling the Holidays

Leading a healthy lifestyle is important, but so is enjoying a busy, full life surrounded by friends and family, celebrating the good times, and supporting one another through the tough ones. Just because you're away from home or attending a family gathering is no reason to feel you won't be able to sustain your commitment to healthy choices. *You will.*

Many lifelong dieters focus on their food fears when they're packing their bags for a cruise or counting the weeks until a relative's wedding. (Well, that and what to wear . . .) Now that you've got the principles of Healthy Exchanges eating down, all you need are a few reminders, some tried-and-true techniques that will keep you focused, and a little encouragement that you're ready to handle the challenges of parties, graduations, family reunions, and that always-dangerous six weeks between Thanksgiving and New Year's . . . which is only a few weeks from the temptation of Valentine's Day candy and Easter baskets!

I'll also show you some great ways for sticking to your HELP lifestyle while you travel (one thing Cliff and I know really well!). Finally, I'll share some tips on how to ask for what you need—in restaurants, from loved ones—and how to get what you want without feeling uncomfortable.

Eating Out with Healthy Exchanges

When I was a professional dieter, I felt safer eating my diet meal at my own table—no distractions or temptations to remind me how deprived I was. And if I was drinking diet shakes or eating prepackaged diet food, I didn't have much of a choice—restaurants were off-limits, and travel was an eating nightmare.

Well, leading a healthy lifestyle might be simpler if we prepared every single meal and snack in the kitchen at home. But that's not my idea of living in the real world—and it's not a way to live for a lifetime!

We don't always eat at home—or have complete control over what we eat. But eating out doesn't have to mean forsaking healthy eating or surrendering to high-fat foods with a shrug. I feel that I know this better than almost anyone else, because I spend so much time on the road. In a recent year, Cliff and I were away from home more than 130 days out of 365, and yet I still managed to lose a couple of pounds instead of gaining a lot more!

What works for me may not be right for you, of course, and I've stressed again and again that HELP is all about finding your own best way to live a healthy life. That said, here are some things I've learned while driving down the interstate on our journeys around the United States.

First, I've found that, when we are driving in the car all day, it works best for me to eat two meals a day, and two snacks. We usually enjoy a late breakfast, an afternoon snack, an early supper, and a snack in the evening. That way, we don't feel bogged down because of our less-active routine.

Our two meals are high in complex carbohydrates and low in fats and sugars. There are so many alternatives nowadays that it's much easier to find healthy choices. I make sure that no two meals

My husband is a minister—need I say more? Church dinners, minister's meetings, house calls with "Oh, just have another one of these cookies" or "Oh, preacher, you must have a piece of this pie or cake—it's my own special recipe." Put them all together, they spell overweight, high blood pressure, and tight clothes.

We began our new way of life in February, and John has already lost thirty-two pounds and I have dropped one and a half sizes in clothes.

—M. M., IA

are exactly alike, because that's how boredom sets in . . . and bad choices follow right behind. Remember, just as you shouldn't spend all your souvenir money at the first place you stop, neither should you use up all your food exchanges at one meal.

I mentioned in the Exercise chapter about our mall walking, which gives us a daily stop to stretch our legs and boost our energy. When we're visiting unfamiliar cities, it's difficult to know which parts of town are safe or unsafe. But we almost always find a shopping mall to walk around in for a couple of miles. Because we consider it a priority, we manage to fit our exercise into each busy day, and we always feel more relaxed when we climb back into the car to head on down the road.

Tactics to Help You Eat Healthily Away from Home

A financial advisor once told me, "People don't plan to fail. They just fail to plan." That applies not only to financial health but also to physical health. It's true that advance planning helps ensure that we stick with our healthy eating program.

When you're eating every meal in a different restaurant, it's easy to feel confused by the variety of selections. If you're feeling a bit fatigued or hungry, you may not be thinking clearly about what choices fit best into your HELP lifestyle.

So let's "prepare" together. I'll share what I've learned as Cliff and I have put thousands of miles on our van over the past five years. I think we've eaten in just about every kind of restaurant, and I've discovered how many ways there are to eat in a healthy way while you're on the road.

Whenever you're eating out, whether it's when you're traveling or just around the corner, it's important to change your focus a bit: concentrate on the conversation and companionship. You'll remember the good time you had much longer than you'll recall how delicious the gravy tasted! And join me in resigning your membership in the Clean Plate Club. I always felt that if I left *anything* on my plate, it was going to waste. After all, I spent good money on that food, and if I didn't eat it, I knew it'd be thrown away.

Well, that *is* one way to look at it. But the truth is this: It's either going to go to waste, or to *your waist*. If you want your dress or pants size to decrease, you have to decrease the amount of food you consume, particularly when eating out.

Don't be ashamed to ask for a doggie bag to be brought to you *at the same time as your meal.* Then, before you eat anything, determine what amount you *should* eat and place the remainder in the doggie bag. Ask the server to keep it for you in the cooler until it's time to call for the check. If you want more than you planned, you're going to have to go back into the kitchen to get it—or ask the server to get it for you. This is a good way to make yourself think twice before overeating. And don't forget, the leftovers can provide a meal or two for another time, so you're saving money as well as calories.

If the restaurant is known for its ample portions, consider sharing an oversized entree with your eating companion. You can still order individual salads, potatoes, rolls, and such. Even if the restaurant charges you extra to do it this way, you'll probably be saving money by not ordering two entrees. And you will feel much better after the meal than if you'd said, "Oh, what the heck! I don't want to cause any fuss; I'll just eat the whole thing myself." Boost your self-esteem and banish those extra inches from your waist by choosing the best way to order *for your health.*

Trust me—if you don't eat it, there is no way your leftovers will go to feed the world's hungry people. Don't fall into that old guilt trip that you're helping others by eating it all yourself. Instead, just eat what you know you should. Then send a check or other donation to a worthwhile charity that will see to it your gift will *really* help feed the hungry.

Now, here are some specific ideas I think you'll find helpful when tackling the challenges of eating out:

- At an all-you-can-eat buffet, walk around the entire buffet before choosing anything. Before a single item goes on your plate, consider all your choices, and decide how to spend your food allowance for the most taste and satisfaction, and the least fat.

- Soup is a great way to satisfy hunger and fill you up. If it's not creamy, cheesy, or fat-laden, I often start with a cup of soup. Good examples include chicken rice or vegetable soup. If the soup contains rice or potatoes, I usually estimate the amount—rarely more than a quarter or half a bread exchange; for most other clear or veggie soups, I count at least

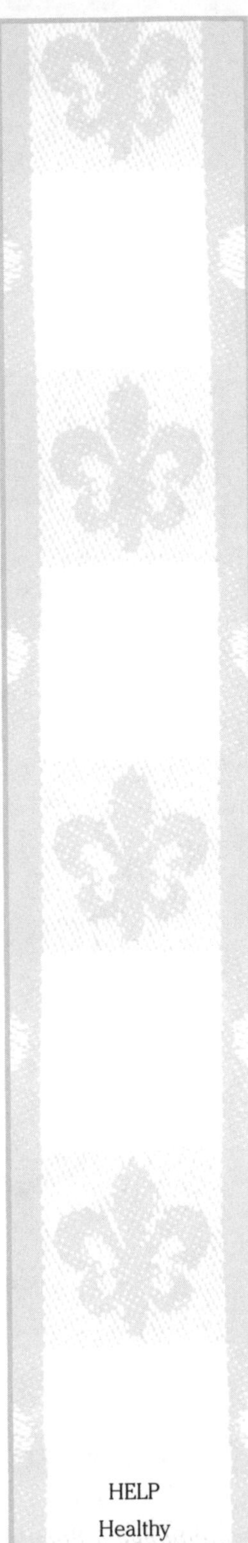

one vegetable exchange, and maybe half of a fat exchange. Let the exchanges fall where they fall!

- If a restaurant or salad bar doesn't have fat-free salad dressing, you have several choices. You can ask for dressing on the side and dip your fork in the dressing before spearing the greens. You'll use much less but still enjoy the taste. Or you can squeeze fresh lemon over the greens to bring out the true flavors of the vegetables (if you've never tried this, it will be a pleasant surprise for you!) or request chunky salsa on the side to spoon over the salad. Toss lightly, and you'll have a fiesta of flavors in your mouth.
- Remember when diets instructed you to have them take the bread basket away, and you sat there feeling deprived and frustrated? Well, I always enjoy a roll when I eat out, but I choose not to have any butter or margarine on it. Most restaurants pride themselves on fresh-baked good bread, and it rarely needs anything on it to improve the taste.
- Read between the lines on the menu. Not everything a restaurant has to offer is listed, and many kitchens are very well stocked with a variety of foods. You wouldn't think twice about asking for a special preparation if you had a medical condition or were allergic to some food. Well, you're eating for your health now, and for enjoyment, too, so it's important to get what you like, prepared the way you need it to be.

I'll Have My "Usual"

Sometimes it's good to have a dish you depend on, no matter where you decide to dine. My "usual" in most restaurants is a baked potato. I didn't always eat potatoes, even with my Irish heritage, because they are high in starch—and for many years were considered "bad" food. Dieters were advised to avoid potatoes like the plague. I even remember using an old "diet" recipe that made "mashed potatoes" from cauliflower.

Talk about a bum rap, though. It wasn't the potato that was bad for us, but the company it kept. Most traditional potato recipes are full of cream, butter, and high-fat cheeses, but the innocent potato was blamed. Now we know better. Potatoes are loaded with vitamins, complex carbohydrates, and potassium. Best of all, they are a low-calorie but tummy-filling food.

I also love to order mashed potatoes, especially at the truck stops Cliff likes to pull into. I order mine plain with a side dish of vegetables, then spoon the vegetables over the potatoes. It's a very tasty and filling addition to whatever small portion of lean protein I'm eating. "Mashed potatoes?" I hear you exclaim. "Aren't they bad for us?" Not really. Remember, the normal restaurant serving is about one-half cup, and the small amount of milk or cream added during preparation is spread throughout the entire container. So enjoy, but say no to topping them with butter or gravy.

I order my potatoes plain, but I *never* eat them that way. After I request that my baked potato be served dry, I also ask for a side dish of fat-free Ranch dressing with a side dish of either salsa or cocktail sauce. I blend a little of the dressing with either and spoon my special "sauce" over the top. Instead of feeling "Poor me!" I savor every bite of that taste sensation. If the restaurant doesn't have fat-free Ranch dressing, I examine the menu until I find something I can use for a topping. Some of my favorite options include: salsa; a side order of vegetables; even a couple of spoonfuls of spaghetti sauce with a light sprinkling of Parmesan cheese. I just do the best I can, *the best I can,* with what is available.

Winning the Breakfast Battle

The more practice you give yourself, the better you'll begin to feel about asking for, and getting, what you want. Breakfast offers lots of healthy choices, but get out of the habit of thinking that dry toast and juice is your best bet—otherwise the feeling of deprivation will drive you straight to the nearest cheese Danish!

Cliff and I eat breakfast out all the time, so I've learned just how many possibilities exist for this start-the-day-off-right meal. Recently we stopped at a small-town cafe for breakfast, and without even looking at the menu I ordered a pancake served without butter. They happened to have a low-calorie maple syrup available, but what I decided to do instead was ask for a serving of fruit cocktail (or any kind of canned fruit). I spooned that on top of the pancake and enjoyed a delicious, fat-free treat. Did I worry if the

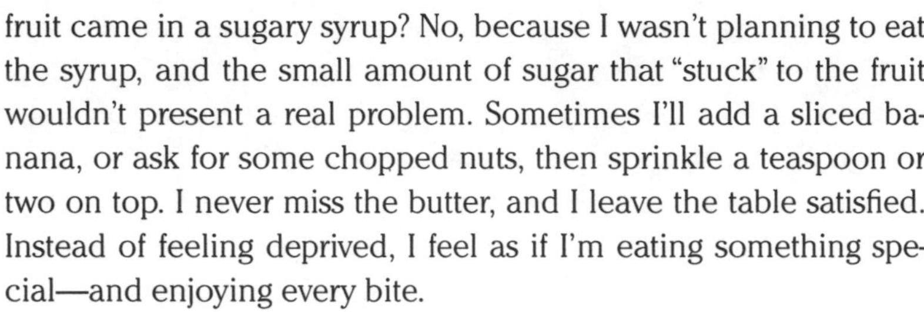

fruit came in a sugary syrup? No, because I wasn't planning to eat the syrup, and the small amount of sugar that "stuck" to the fruit wouldn't present a real problem. Sometimes I'll add a sliced banana, or ask for some chopped nuts, then sprinkle a teaspoon or two on top. I never miss the butter, and I leave the table satisfied. Instead of feeling deprived, I feel as if I'm eating something special—and enjoying every bite.

In the colder months, I often like to order oatmeal (without cream, of course) and a small container of jelly. I stir the jelly into the hot oatmeal and savor every bite. I could also stir some low-calorie maple syrup and a spoonful of walnuts into the cereal and enjoy a dish as tasty as any on the menu!

Another good breakfast option is asking for a plain baking-powder biscuit, a side dish of any canned fruit, and a small glass of skim milk. I ask that the biscuit be served in a cereal bowl. When my order arrives, I spoon the fruit over the biscuit and pour a small amount of the milk over the top. It's almost like eating shortcake for breakfast!

My "usual" is a veggie omelet made with egg substitutes if they have them. If they don't, I ask them to use one whole egg and several egg whites, plus any vegetables they have on hand. The other day, I ordered a veggie omelet in a rustic truck stop, was happy to find they had egg substitutes, and enjoyed a "three-egg" omelet stuffed with chopped broccoli, celery, onions, tomatoes, and mushrooms, with just one slice of cheese on top. Sometimes I skip the cheese and ask for salsa on the side to spoon over the top. Omelets aren't just for breakfast, either. I often order one for lunch or dinner and enjoy every bite.

And it's not written in stone that you must eat traditional breakfast foods for breakfast. Let your imagination roam when you're studying the menu, then order whatever strikes your fancy as long as it's low fat and low sugar. If pasta with vegetables or a baked potato piques your interest, and it's available, go for it. Your taste buds will thank you for the wake-up call!

Adding South-of-the-Border Spice

Do you love to eat at Mexican restaurants as much as I do but find yourself filling up on sour cream, guacamole, and the entire basket of chips? You don't have to deny yourself the pleasure of dining out on this spicy cuisine, but having a few fat-saving secrets will help you stick with your plan to eat healthily. Some restaurants (including the chains Chi-Chi's and Ruby Tuesdays) will prepare a fat-free veggie fajita if you request it when you order. They will gladly grill the veggies in tomato juice, and you can ask them to add chicken, shrimp, or steak as well. Just request that they leave the sour cream and guacamole off your plate—and to bring *extra* salsa! Then when the fajita and fixin's arrive, spoon lettuce, tomatoes, and sizzling veggies into your tortillas, drizzle salsa over the top, and enjoy every mouthwatering bite. If these national chains will take the extra trouble to give a regular customer what she wants, I bet your local restaurants will be happy to do it too.

What about those chips? Some people can ignore the basket even if it's placed right in front of them, but others, like me, are easily tempted. How do I handle this without depriving myself of a taste I enjoy? I count out six chips as a bread choice and place them in front of me. I take my time eating these with generous dips into the bowl of salsa. I know that when they are gone, I'm finished with the chips. Instead of just reaching into the basket and eating without thinking, I've chosen to enjoy this treat in moderation. The first few times it may be hard to stick with your planned portion, but you'll probably find it gets easier each time you do it.

So, the next time the family says, "Let's eat Mexican tonight," be the first in the car. You can enjoy a fiesta of spicy tastes without overloading on fat—and you won't have to do the dishes!

Chinese If You Please

Chinese food is another great Healthy Exchanges option, but it's important to be aware of how some of your favorite dishes are prepared. Just because a dish includes lots of vegetables doesn't mean it's healthy. The secret is usually in the sauce.

Recently we went to a Chinese restaurant, and I said no to the buffet, because there were too many things there that can grab you when you're hungry. Instead I ordered off the menu. Many Chinese dishes rely on lots of vegetables with very little protein, cooked quickly to retain nutrients. (Stir-frying is a great cooking method and uses very little oil.) Broccoli with chicken, beef, or

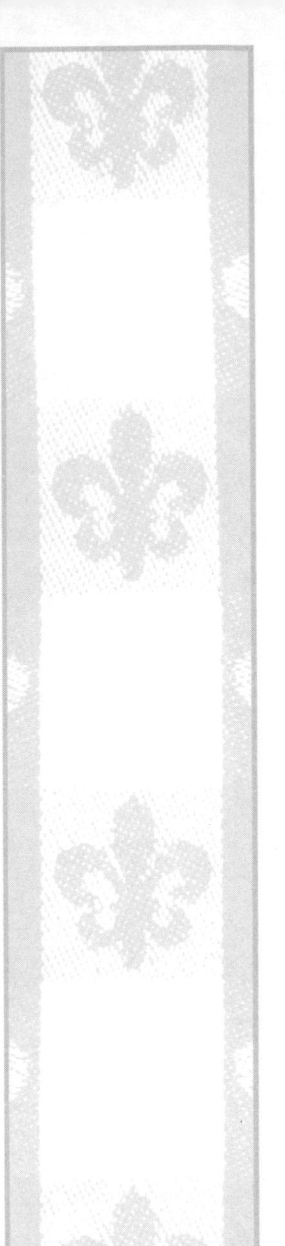

pork, or shrimp with vegetables are some of my favorites. (Cliff passed on all these—he hates broccoli and won't eat shrimp under any circumstances!) We eat our rice steamed instead of fried and often order Won Ton or Hot and Sour Soup.

Just try to stay away from dishes that are prepared with a lot of oil, like Fried Rice, Egg Rolls, Sweet and Sour Pork, Fried Won Tons, and Crispy Fried Beef. (That "Fried" is a definite giveaway, isn't it?)

Yes, you can read *and* eat your fortune cookie. One has about 19 calories and almost no fat. It counts as ½ Starch for diabetics. I hope your fortune reads: *Good Friends, Good Food, and Good Health Ahead.*

Bring on the Pasta!

Italian restaurants hardly need a special section in this chapter, as they offer so many possibilities for delicious and healthy dining. Just a few cautionary notes before you dine *en Italiano*: Skip the olive oil often offered these days as a dip for that wonderfully crusty Italian bread; while it's healthier than other fats, it's still 100 percent fat! As a terrific alternative, I often order a couple of fresh-baked breadsticks served *dry,* along with a side dish of marinara sauce for dipping. Mmmmm—very low fat and very good!

Then, if my salad comes topped with butter-soaked croutons, I just push them aside. I prefer the breadsticks as both a healthier and tastier alternative. An important part of healthy dining out is recognizing that you have to pick and choose. You *can't* have it all—but you can enjoy some of the best a restaurant has to offer.

For your entree, choose any of the *delicioso* red sauces over your choice of pasta, from angel hair to fusilli twists, or perhaps a fresh clam sauce. But be careful about sauces that shade from pink to white—their main ingredient is cream! You're generally better off enjoying creamy pasta sauces at home, where you can work magic with Healthy Exchanges recipes that call for evaporated skim milk or Healthy Request soups.

Just Desserts

I usually steer clear of the dessert bar or menu when I'm eating out, or else I order fresh berries or melon. I know that restaurant desserts are much higher in fat and sugar than my own "sinful-looking but sinless" creations. With all the Healthy Exchanges pie and cake desserts I get at home, I don't find it hard to pass when it's time for dessert at a restaurant.

Of course, I occasionally do decide to enjoy a dessert on the road. I try to make sure it's either as healthy as it can be, or that it is a special treat I can't find anywhere else. Some healthy desserts I enjoy out include: "ice cream" at a TCBY parlor, any fresh fruit in season, and strawberry shortcake without the whipped cream or ice cream.

My true special treat is *real* bread pudding. Since it's rarely available on the menu, I don't end up ordering it very often. When I do succumb to that "dessert of all desserts," I savor the first bite, relish the second, and enjoy the third bite slowly. Then I throw my napkin over the rest and call it quits. Those few bites are enough to keep me happy and content—and my waistline doesn't have to suffer the consequences of overdoing it.

High-fat and sugar-laden desserts are the downfall of many, but they don't have to spell disaster for you. Pick out your times and selections carefully and enjoy what you choose to the fullest. Life without any dessert is dull and boring, but life with too many desserts is unhealthy and fattening.

A Thirst for Good Health

My beverage of choice at home or eating out has always been water—and that's water without the slice of lemon, please. If I want lemonade, then I'll order lemonade. When I request water, it's the cold, clear taste of plain water I want. Cliff has always referred to me as a "cheap date" because of my beverage choice. In fact, he often tells the server just to "leave the pitcher" because it'll save so much running back and forth as I empty my glass again and again.

I order water because I love the icy taste of it. But I'm glad to know that by drinking it I'm doing my body a favor. Most people don't drink nearly enough water on any given day. I, on the other hand, drink at least eight to twelve glasses of water every day. And no, I'm not excusing myself to go to the ladies' room every fifteen minutes.

I know that many people resist drinking lots of water because they believe it will add water weight and they'll feel bloated. In fact, the opposite is true. If you don't drink enough water, your body tends to retain the little you do consume so your tissues can maintain a fluid balance. It's ironic, isn't it, but the more water you drink, the less water retention you will experience. More good news: Your body will soon adjust to finally getting enough of that liquid nectar it depends on. After the first several days, you won't be running to the bathroom all the time.

I like to think that one of the reasons my face doesn't betray the fact that I'm over fifty or that I've lost 130 pounds is that I've always kept my skin moisturized with the natural "fountain of youth," water. Water does more for your complexion than the most expensive facial cream on the market. If you find it hard to drink water for the benefits your body derives from it, try thinking of it as the ultimate wrinkle eraser! Now, doesn't that make the water taste better already?

Eating What You Want—and Only What You Want

I give myself a signal when I've had enough food. In the old days, the signal that I'd had enough was that the plate was empty and I would stop eating. Now, when I think I'm starting to get to that feeling of comfortable fullness, I crumple up my napkin and put it on my plate. Regardless of what's left on the plate, I'm done. Once I do that, it's just a matter of moments before a server picks up the plate and takes it away. And it makes it harder for you to remove the napkin and go on eating what you already decided you shouldn't have.

Some people sprinkle a bunch of salt or pepper on the food once they've decided they've had enough. You could ask to take the extra portion home, but you don't have to. And you don't have to worry if the chef is insulted that you didn't finish. It's how *you* feel—your health—that's important.

Another thing I never do anymore is live "artificially." That means I never take food into the restaurant with me. Never! I make do with whatever's there. That's what real people do. I don't allow those little diet crutches into my life anymore. We went out for lunch at a restaurant recently that offered a grilled Italian chicken breast sandwich, but didn't have any fat-free dressing on hand. I asked them to bring me some chunky salsa and some shrimp cocktail sauce, and I mixed my own fat-free dressing. I feel even something as minor as bringing salad dressing to a restaurant is a crutch, like a pacifier to a baby. I'll use it at home if I choose; I'll order it if the restaurant offers it; but if they don't, I prefer to improvise the best I can when I eat out. It's part of my decision to live like a normal person—and part of my positive attitude that I can make decisions based on what's available. What happens that one time when you don't have the diet dressing with you? Because you haven't prepared to handle the situation, you may feel "Why bother?" and opt for something full of fat and calories.

Cliff would probably fall off his chair if I went into a restaurant and ordered my meal "as is," without tailoring my order to exactly what I want to eat. In the movie *When Harry Met Sally*, Meg Ryan got a lot of laughs by doing just the same. She simply wanted her food *the way she wanted it*—so she patiently asked for it that way every time.

It's not necessary to be difficult or aggressive about your requests. Instead, be assertive. Explain clearly how you would like your food to be served, and ask for what's reasonably available. The other day we pulled into a truck stop that was featuring roast pork sandwiches with mashed potatoes and gravy. I ordered it, but asked the waitress to hold the gravy and bring me a roll instead of the two slices of bread. I also requested cooked vegetables, and they were happy to substitute cooked carrots for the gravy. I enjoyed a meal that was almost like a pork pot roast without most of the usual fat. All because *I wasn't afraid to ask.*

Make sure you're living in the real world, though. Don't go into McDonald's and ask for a baked potato—they don't offer one on their menu. You need to know when you go into a fast-food restaurant what your options are.

In general, though, there are few places that aren't going to try to give you what you want, *within reason*. They want the server to get a tip, they want you to tell everyone what a great place it is, and they want you to come back. It's just sound business practice.

Happiness is contagious . . . be a carrier!

—A. O., IL

Anyplace that is too snooty or rigid to do what you want doesn't deserve your business anyway. So don't give them your hard-earned money.

If you order your food one way and it comes another way, you need only say in a nice way, I believe I ordered it such-and-such and that's how I need it. Or that's how I want it. The few times this has happened to me, they couldn't have been nicer. They whisked it away and brought me exactly what I wanted with no fuss whatsoever.

Do you find yourself thinking, "I don't want to make a fuss"? or that you don't want everyone else to have to wait for you? But ask yourself this: Who's really paying for the food in the long run? You're paying twice—paying money for food you didn't want and you're paying for it healthwise.

Above all, *don't stay home*, thinking that if you're not faced with temptation you won't give in. Enjoying a good restaurant meal with friends and family is one of the pleasures of life, and you can learn to cope. Besides, eating out means you don't have to do the dishes!

TRAVELING WITH HELP

When you're planning a cruise or other vacation, pack your positive attitude along with your swimsuit and other vacation gear—and you will do just fine. While many people warn you that a cruise is just a "floating buffet table" and that you're bound to return home five to ten pounds heavier than when you departed, I can promise you a wonderful time on your holiday, and one that doesn't mean gaining weight through overeating.

Cliff and I went on a cruise a few years ago to celebrate our wedding anniversary, so I know firsthand about the food available at all hours of the day and night. But I walked off that ship without having gained a pound. Here are some of the ideas that worked for me.

First, know your limitations. You can't eat six full meals and four snacks every day, no matter where you are. Don't eat all your food choices in one meal, but spread them out during the day.

Most cruise lines offer lighter fare highlighted on their menus. And just as you would at home, try to choose a variety of foods during the course of the cruise. Enjoy fish one day, chicken the next, and lean beef for another evening. Limit your alcohol intake. (You usually pay for alcohol, so that may help you to go lightly on the champagne.)

Do make sure you attend at least one midnight buffet. You have to, just to gaze in wonder at the ice sculptures. But think carefully about eating a high-fat dessert at that late hour. A better choice might be a beautiful piece of exotic fresh fruit.

After your meals, why not make it a habit to take a stroll on the deck. It feels absolutely wonderful to walk in the fresh air with the sea breeze blowing and nothing but ocean as far as the eye can see. Take the day excursions offered when you're in port—and walk, walk, walk! One of my fondest memories is hiking up a "mountain" in Jamaica, then walking in a stream on the way back down. And while you're on the ship, enjoy as many activities as possible—aerobic classes, dancing in the nightclub, reading by the pool, having a massage. Before you know it, your vacation will be over—and you'll be home with great memories, and no extra pounds!

Here's one last suggestion for a bit of a "reality check" while you're away. We usually dress for comfort and ease when we're on vacation, in shorts or slacks with elastic waists. I recommend that, at least a couple of days a week, you wear clothing with a real waistband. If you don't, you may not realize until you get home that your waistline went on vacation, too! If you discover that your clothes feel a little tighter than when you started your journey, you may think twice before saying yes to second helpings!

Healthy Flying

I learned a long time ago to place an order for a special meal when I make airplane reservations. Because I want low fat and low sugar, I always ask for the diabetic meal. You can also order a fresh fruit plate, a low-fat meal, even vegetarian. These special meals are always the best, in my opinion—not bland and boring like many airline low-cal meals, just low sugar and reasonably low fat. I often notice my neighbors looking at my plate with envy, and I can tell they're thinking, "Now, why didn't I think to order that?" The meal almost always includes fresh fruit for dessert along with the healthy entree.

As long as you give the airline at least twenty-four hours, you should be able to arrange a special meal, so remember to ask your travel agent to order it the next time you plan to travel. You truly can eat and enjoy healthy food while flying. Best of all, your good intentions won't *fly away* when the meal is placed in front of you!

Skip the peanuts if they're offered, but if you're truly hungry, munch on those low-fat pretzels. Of course, if you don't take them, you won't eat them—and you'll quickly forget about them. Instead, enjoy a glass of ice water, a diet soda, or some orange or tomato juice. Then, have a healthy snack after you land at your destination.

Snacking and Eating on the Run

It's important not to let yourself get hungry, because you've either skipped meals or not planned to eat for too long. We all really know our own bodies better than anyone else does. I really get upset and irate with diet plans that dare to tell you when you can and when you cannot eat. We all have different time clocks, and I know for a fact that no matter what I had for lunch—it can be the tiniest of meals, or the biggest feast—come 4:30, I'm hungry. Cliff looks at me as if I were literally crazy because I want to have a snack then. But every evening about 8:30 *he* wants something to munch on—and he wants it to be crunchy—before he goes to bed.

You may be surprised to hear that I don't keep an "emergency kit" in the car or van with us, but there's always somewhere to stop. We've pulled into truck stops, we've stopped in mom-and-pop diners, fast-food restaurants, and convenience stores. There's always something somewhere. I think that people who say they have no options are really fooling themselves. The choices are there, but *you* have to make them.

Cliff likes to eat pretzels, and if he picks up the reduced-sodium kind, I'll have some too. Generally, though, I don't like salty things, so I tend to zero in on fresh fruit and reduced-fat crackers. (You have to be careful when you've got the entire box of crackers in the car, though; it's too easy to keep munching until the box is empty!) One food I'm careful to avoid snacking on: muffins. They're usually so high in fat and sugar, you could easily consume three-fourths of your day's worth of fat grams by eating just one.

I also drink lots of water when we travel, and I enjoy Diet Mountain Dew too.

Enjoy your snacks, just as you enjoy your meals. They're an important part of not feeling deprived or on a restricted diet. Many nutritionists suggest eating smaller meals more often, to aid digestion and keep blood sugar stable. So, no matter where you are—at home or on the go—plan for healthy snacks that will satisfy your hunger and give your taste buds a wonderful time.

It is the greatest of all mistakes to do nothing because you can do only a little. Do what you can.

—Sydney Smith

You're Not Helpless during the Holidays

Are you wondering how you're going to make it through the "Holiday Binge Season"? You've been invited to lots of parties, you're having your own tree-trimming celebration, and you know you'll be cooking for company more than once. What should you do?

You're not alone in your concern. But by taking a positive approach to this beautiful time of the year, when we make a special effort to show our love and generosity to others through our actions, you can face the challenge of the holidays with a smile—and a dazzling selection of Healthy Exchanges treats guaranteed to rival those on any table.

It's your decision, of course. Will you tell yourself that this season comes but once a year, and by golly you're going to enjoy every minute, and every bite? Or will you decide to take it one day at a time and do your best to make healthy choices? For many of us, the holiday season is a combination of the two.

What are some techniques that will make it easier to handle the abundance of high-fat foods that confront you everywhere you go? Most of us attend more family get-togethers, social celebrations, and company holiday parties between Thanksgiving and New Year's Day than at any other time of the year. You can count on food being the first invited guest to all of them. The national average is to gain about ten pounds during this short holiday season—but you don't have to be part of that depressing statistic!

You can enjoy the season and not watch your waistline grow—I promise. All it takes is a little preplanning *before* the parties are in full swing. And that *doesn't* include the option of hiding at home, trying to avoid temptation. Living healthily means living life to the fullest, not adhering to a rigid plan that doesn't allow for any of life's extras.

It really helps to know your options in advance so you can plan your daily food choices accordingly.

- Are you going to a family potluck or shared-dish dinner? Then why not take food you *know* is tasty, filling, and healthy?
- If it is a sit-down dinner, can you offer to "help the host out" by bringing something? Of course, that something you bring will be an attractive Healthy Exchanges dish *you* can eat with confidence because you know it's healthy!

I'll bet that other guests will appreciate your "something" also.

Make sure you always have plenty of healthy holiday snacks on hand. Fat-free pretzels, yogurt-based dips, and refreshing cranberry punches are all good presents of food for you and others. *You* are worth the little extra effort to have traditional foods of the season around. Just make sure you prepare them the Healthy Exchanges way. You never know when unexpected family or Christmas carolers will drop in. It's much better to bring out the healthy treats you already have prepared than to run out for pizza and ice cream to serve your company. It's also more economical.

Partying with Pleasure

How about eating one of those healthy snacks and drinking lots of water before you head out the door to party at someone else's home? A filling snack *really* does take the edge off your appetite and enables you to choose the food and beverages you can enjoy much more wisely when you arrive at the party. Your brain will be making the choices, not your empty stomach. I think you may be

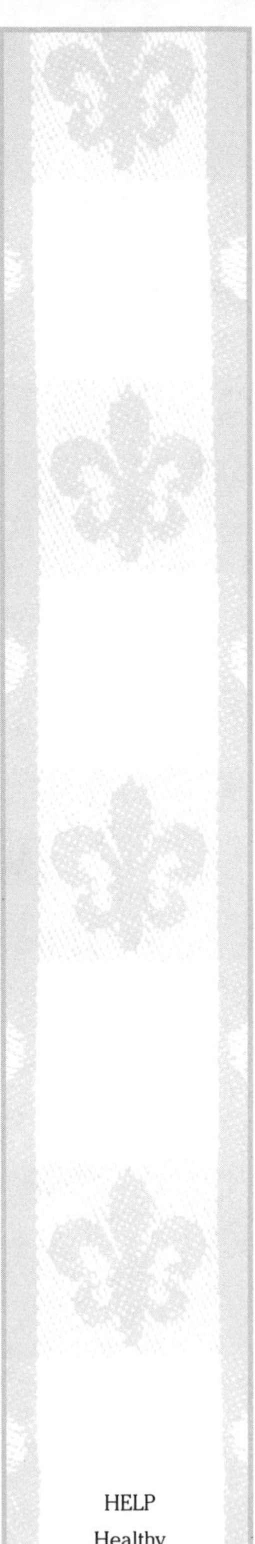

surprised at how much more selective you are when your appetite has been checked along with your coat.

When you arrive at the party or social event, scope out the room before doing anything else. Where are the guests congregating? Is there a buffet table? Where is the bar? It's a good idea to sit as far away from the food as possible, so you are not just grabbing food because it's "handy." Concentrate on visiting with friends instead. When you do go to the buffet table, look everything over once before putting anything on your plate. Then, fill your plate with *the best choices available*, and walk away. Eat your food as slowly as possible and *don't* go back for seconds. You may regret not eating "all those cookies" for a moment or two when you see others consuming them by the handful, but by the time you are ready to call it an evening, you will be glad you *just said no.*

If you are not the designated driver, and you want to partake of the liquid "holiday sunshine," choose to drink only one or two glasses of holiday spirits, and sip them slowly. Remember that alcohol is nothing but empty calories that react in your body just the way fat does. If you choose not to drink and don't want people pushing alcoholic beverages on you all night long, ask for a diet soda mixed with club soda and garnish it with a slice of lime. Hold that glass in your hand at all times. It'll keep people from asking if you need a refill and guarantee your hands will be so busy that it's more difficult to reach for potato chips or other tempting snacks that happen to be sitting around.

If you will be attending a catered company Christmas party and don't have a choice about the food being served, you may be eating foods you would otherwise not have chosen. *Just make the best of the situation.* No one said you *had* to eat everything on your plate! Select carefully from what is put in front of you. Remind yourself that you don't eat like this every day, and so it's not necessary to make a big fuss over the food. Before putting one bite into your mouth, though, decide how much of whatever is on your plate you "should" eat, and then enjoy every bite of *that much.* Take the fork and slowly stir the rest around a bit, then put your napkin over the plate to signal to yourself that you're finished eating. If you play it low-key, most people won't realize that you aren't eating everything and won't make a big deal out of it. It's only when you announce that you're on a diet, then eat everything in sight when the food comes—rationalizing that it's a "once-a-year special event"—that people wonder about your eating habits and even make jokes about them.

You have time for anything you decide to make time for!

—D. A., IA

"Earning" a Few Extras

For any occasion when you know that you will be eating more because of "social obligations," why not plan to do a little more exercise *the day of* and *the day after* the big event? Walk an extra mile or two. Then you can "spend" those calories (you've earned them!) at the special event, without feeling guilty. But remember, if you decide to put in those extra miles, you have to follow through and DO IT. Don't just think about it. The road to big hips is paved with good intentions!

Making a special effort to schedule time for moderate exercise will help get you through the hectic weeks of shopping and preparing for company. Not only will it de-stress you, it will remind you how far you've come already and strengthen your resolve to make the best choices you can. The HELP lifestyle is flexible enough to incorporate special occasions, and if Thanksgiving just isn't a holiday without your mother's sweet-potato pie, then have a piece—but maybe add fifteen minutes to your walk the next morning!

With a healthy outlook about holiday events, you can enjoy the season—and still feel good about yourself and your commitment to healthy living habits. Only you can decide if you're going to beat the odds or become a casualty of the "Holiday Binge Season." Because you're not on a diet, but living a healthy way of life, you can handle the holidays . . . and the rest of the year, too.

Whether you're the host or the guest, focus on visiting with friends more than on the holiday foods. It's a good idea to remind yourself that the holidays aren't just about food, although it's definitely one of the pleasures of the season. But it's also a great time to reconnect with friends you haven't seen in a while, show off photos of your grandchildren (it's practically impossible to eat when you've got your hands full of pictures that you don't want to get greasy!), and enjoy basking in the compliments you're sure to receive as friends and family get a look at the new you. You may find yourself sharing your "secret" all evening long—and discover it's time to go home before you've even located the dessert table!

And if you should "stray," remember that one or two lapses do NOT mean a collapse of your healthy lifestyle. Don't let occasional episodes of overeating ruin your positive attitude. Congratulate yourself on your progress so far—and keep up the good work!

Handling Comments on Your Success

Let me say just a few words here about an unexpected challenge you may experience during the holidays, and in the weeks and months ahead, as you progress on the HELP plan. People will very probably tell you how good you look—something you haven't heard in a while, perhaps. If you're like many people who've struggled with their weight over the years, you've heard both positive and negative comments, and both may make you equally uncomfortable.

Maybe someone comes up to you and says, "Congratulations—you look great tonight!" Your first impulse may be to demur, even to disagree: "Oh, it's only ten pounds" or "No, really, I didn't lose an ounce this week." Learn how to take a compliment. Say "thank you." Say, "I feel great, and that's what's really important to me." Smile and accept the wonderful gift of warmth being offered to you.

Perhaps others with less tact may comment, "You've lost weight again, haven't you? Do you think you'll keep it off this time?" They may have recognized your success but at the same moment tapped into your fears about sustaining your weight loss. (Don't you just want to dump a pitcher of eggnog over their heads?) It's best not to answer a question like this—it can only lead to debate and squelch any possible holiday spirit you have left. I suggest you look them in the eye, just say, "Thanks, I'm feeling really good. Would you excuse me—I see someone I must talk to!" and scram!

The holidays are a time of intense emotion, and they often trigger old, unhealthy eating behaviors you've worked hard to leave behind you. By practicing your responses, by choosing how you want to feel during this time, you'll be able to carry your positive attitude through the season and celebrate more than you ever expected!

I've cooked at home more in the last month and a half than in the nine years I've been married. Your recipes are truly an answer to a prayer!

—K. S., NM

When Showing Love Means Sharing Food

Going home for the holidays can present an abundance of challenges for someone who's chosen a healthy lifestyle. Does your mom make a fuss if you don't eat everything special she prepares "just for you"? If she doesn't get to see you very often, she may look forward all year to "fussing over" you when you come home for Christmas. But how can you stick with your healthy eating plan *and* not hurt her feelings when she shows love by preparing all that food?

This is a real dilemma—not just a food quandary but an emotional one as well. Many parents show their love for us by preparing our favorite foods, sometimes because they can't say they love us in words or hugs. When my daughter, Becky, comes home, I always want to show my love by making her favorite, Becky's Southern Banana Pecan Cream Pie. But now I fix that pie and all her other favorites the Healthy Exchanges way.

Here's one solution that may work for you. Think about the types of foods that your mother always wants to make "just for you." Then hunt up some healthy recipes that are similar in taste, texture, and aroma. Call or write your mother that you are trying to lose weight, or lower your cholesterol, or stabilize your blood sugar, and that you really need her help when you come home. Tell her that you have found some recipes that aren't quite as good as hers but that are lower in fat and sugar, and that you would love to help her prepare them. Ask her if she will wait until you get there so you can go to the store together and shop for what you need to make the dishes. Then ask her if the two of you could have a private "party" in the kitchen trying out the new recipes. I can almost guarantee your mother will be thrilled to think that the two of you will be sharing quality time together, and she'll cooperate. Once she sees that you still want the love that the food allows her to give you, she probably won't mind that the actual recipes are healthier versions of family favorites. It's the giving process that matters most to her anyway. Maybe you'll "cook up" some new favorite dishes together and help your entire family eat healthily.

A Healthy Lifestyle Doesn't Mean Family Favorites Are Off-limits

One of my subscribers recently shared with me the happy news of her thirty-pound weight loss but confessed she was nervous about heading home for a family reunion potluck. She felt great about her new shape but was worried about handling the temptation of all those special family dishes she still loves but doesn't eat anymore.

I believe it's a question of setting priorities long before you arrive at the reunion. Are there a few extra-special dishes you know will show up on the party table, dishes you just can't get anywhere else and that are truly a part of your family's traditions? If there are—and there usually are—then plan to savor a reasonable serving of these unique foods. Enjoy them, *without fear*, and *in moderation.*

But be sure to pass on those foods you can have anytime and anywhere. They're just not "special" enough for this special occasion. Put your personal favorites on your plate, then find a place to sit as far from the food table as possible. Remind yourself that you're not going back for seconds, and focus on the best part of family reunions—*the family*. Visit with those loved ones you haven't seen in so long, catch up on family news, and share your own.

Be sure to ooh and aah over every bite you choose to enjoy, and tell Aunt Sarah that her apple crisp (or whatever) is just as delicious as you remembered. If she presses you to have another piece, thank her for her generosity—but say you've really had enough for now. "Maybe later," you might add if she's disappointed. (It doesn't mean you have to, but it usually ends the discussion for the moment.) And if you're leaving the party, and she packs a care package full of goodies for you, accept it with a smile. You can share it with friends at work on Monday—or put it in the freezer to save for another special time.

Enjoy the compliments you get on your new figure and healthy complexion. If you're asked, tell people why you look and feel so good. You're setting a great example for younger family members by showing that beloved family food traditions can have a place in a healthy lifestyle—as long as they're savored in moderation.

Success consists of getting up just one more time than you fall.

—Anonymous

Nine

Hitting a Plateau . . . or Falling Off the Health Wagon

Every dieter has had the frustrating experience of getting stuck, of reaching a period of days or weeks during which weight loss stops or slows and fear sets in: Is this as far as I can go? Am I about to start backsliding and regain the weight? *Why isn't it working anymore?*

So many people have confided in me that they feel like failures because they lost weight, sometimes a lot of weight—and then almost overnight the weight loss stopped. No matter what they did—living on lettuce, never eating after 4 P.M., giving up salt—they couldn't get the needle on the scale to move!

They were devastated, thinking that they *must* have done something wrong because the rest just wouldn't come off. And they were impatient, too, counting the days until the weight was off and the diet was over. They wanted to lose it all as quickly as possible, had even plotted out how long a particular number of pounds would take to lose—and now the schedule was ruined.

I know the feeling well.

I experienced *many* plateaus during the time it took me to lose 130 pounds. Most of us have experienced the plateaus that are a part of every weight-loss program. You may not now share my unique philosophy that they exist for a purpose, but I hope you'll keep an open mind. And if you're looking for ways to "climb back on" the Health Wagon after you've fallen off, I'll try to help you pick up where you left off instead of starting all over again.

When you flee temptation, be sure not to leave a forwarding address.

When "Disaster" Strikes . . .

Everything's been going so well. You've been following the HELP plan for weeks or months now—eating healthy, delicious meals with your family, making time for regular, moderate exercise, changing old habits for new healthy ones, and keeping your spirits high with a positive attitude. You've lost weight, lowered your cholesterol, gotten your blood sugar under control, and suddenly—

The scale is stuck on the same number.

Your clothes aren't getting any looser.

Instead of looking forward to your workouts, you've been feeling exhausted, your body sluggish.

WHAT'S WRONG????????

You've probably hit the "evil" plateau, the bane of every dieter's existence. It feels as if the motor has died, the car has stalled, and the future that looked so bright and hopeful is suddenly cloudy and gray.

WELL, DON'T BELIEVE IT.

When I talk to groups of people, I always hear them groan when I bring up this subject. And they groan even louder when, instead of sympathizing or offering some secret method to avoid plateaus, I challenge their expectations—and say that I believe plateaus are God's gift to the body.

What? How is that possible? How can a plateau be a good thing?

When I speak of the journey we're taking together as part of the HELP blueprint for success, I often liken it to a cross-country car trip. (Maybe I see it this way because I'm married to Cliff, who covered just about every mile of the United States before he gave up long-haul trucking and started hauling me around!)

If you traveled nonstop from New York to Los Angeles, driving all by yourself, you'd arrive exhausted both physically and emotionally. Your body would be a wreck, and it might take days or weeks to recover your energy and health.

But if you stopped along the way—maybe as often as every few hundred miles or so—took a shower, relaxed over a good meal, slept a few hours in a comfortable bed, you'd arrive at your destination in great shape. And you'd have enjoyed the trip in a way you never would have if you'd driven the entire way without pausing to refresh yourself.

Maybe I'm stretching the image a little, but I think a plateau works much the same way. By stopping for just a bit, your body has a chance to catch up to the changes that have been occurring inside and out over the past weeks. Your skin has the opportunity to shrink along with your waist, so you won't look like "death warmed over" as you get closer to your goal weight. I think it even gives the brain a chance to catch up to the body, so that the new habits you've been teaching your body become a part of how you see yourself and how you act.

Often, after a very quick weight loss, the body may be wearing a smaller size dress or slacks, but the mind is still in the "large sizes." You need the plateau time to practice thinking and acting like a thin person, getting used to a "steady as she goes" way of life instead of the yo-yo, up-and-down, on-and-off approach of the professional dieter.

Trying to rush things is a symptom of the way you used to live—a way you've decided not to anymore. If your primary goal has always been to lose weight quickly so you can get back to living the way you did before, it's time to focus on a different one. A plateau can be a kind of reminder that you shouldn't set a time limit on living a healthy life. HELP is a lifetime plan, not something to try for a few weeks or months. *Stick with it, or your weight will stick with you.*

Plateaus don't last forever, and once your body has a chance to rest, it will continue the journey forward. Just keep doing what you've been doing, and you'll soon start to see measurable results again.

Should you do anything different when you're stuck on a plateau? No. And yes. No, you should continue following your program of healthy eating, exercise, goal setting, and keeping a positive attitude. But yes, use this "reminder" to do a mental Reality Check.

- Are you making time to prepare healthy and appealing foods instead of depriving yourself in hopes you'll lose weight faster?
- Are you drinking at least eight glasses of water every day?
- Are you fitting a session of moderate exercise into your life four to five times each week and keeping track of your accomplishments?
- Are you rewarding yourself for reaching mini-goals and setting new ones regularly?
- Are you still writing in your Positive Actions diary and rereading it when you feel frustrated?

If you are doing all you can—*the best you can*—then keep up the good work! The pounds will start coming off again soon, but in the meantime, make sure you're enjoying your life to the fullest.

You may be disappointed if you fail, but you are doomed if you don't try.

—Beverly Sills

Falling Off the "Health Wagon"

But what if the plateau has discouraged you so much that you've started skipping your exercise sessions? Maybe you got so angry at the scale you hid it in the closet and said, "The heck with it. If I'm not losing weight, why should I keep eating this way, when I'd kill for a juicy burger and fries?" Perhaps you've even gained back a few pounds by letting your new healthy habits slide. Or what if you feel you've followed the plan to the letter and still gained a pound or two!

STOP. Take a deep breath and blow it out. Take another one.

It's not too late to pick up where you left off, no matter how you've "strayed." Start right now—by writing down what you've already eaten today and what you're planning to eat for the rest of the day. Decide to fit in some exercise *today*, even if it's just a fifteen-minute walk. Remind yourself of what you wanted when you started the Healthy Exchanges Lifetime Plan, and ask yourself if those goals still matter to you.

If they do—and I believe they will—then do *one* thing that

points you on your journey to good health again. Buy some fresh vegetables at the grocery store for a salad; toss that half-empty bag of chips into the nearest trash can. Say out loud, "Nobody's perfect." Say, "Nobody's perfect, but I can live healthily one day at a time."

Instead of filling your head with negative self-talk, give yourself credit for what you've already accomplished. Think about where you might be if you hadn't followed the HELP plan for the past weeks or months. If you find yourself muttering that you've *only* lost five pounds so far, take a quick trip to the grocery store and pick up five pounds of butter in the dairy case. Think how good it feels not to be carrying around that weight anymore. (If butter isn't convincing, try a five-pound roasting chicken, or a bag of kitty litter. Don't you feel the weight off your hips now?)

If you find yourself frustrated by having gained back some of the weight you lost, if you feel bad about having to "do it again," you're living in the past. *You don't have to anymore*. Look forward, renew your commitment to a healthy lifestyle for a lifetime, and resolve to take better care of yourself.

Now grab my hand and find a seat on the Health Wagon here beside me and the rest of us human beings. We may not be perfect, but we can do better today than we did yesterday.

Handling Negative People

Have you got some old eating buddies? You know, those friends who shared your donut or pizza binges, who encouraged you to join them for a sundae you didn't really want but agreed to gobble down?

Most of us have them, and here's one thing I've learned over the past few years: *You usually don't convert them*. You can talk all you want about your choice to live healthily, but I think it's wrong to try to ram it down their throats.

I've never been able to stand opinionated people who think their way is the *only* way. These people seem to think that you must agree with their solutions, whether the topic is healthy food or politics. I just don't believe in forcing what I believe on anyone else.

If people want to embrace my philosophy, that's great, and I'll help all I can. If they choose to follow a totally different lifestyle, that's *their choice*.

I never, ever do "plate patrol." *Never*. What you put on your plate, and in your mouth, is your personal decision. What I put on my plate and in my mouth is my personal decision. If you happen to want to put the same thing on your plate and in your mouth as I do, that's great. But if you choose something different, I won't interfere. It's your life—and your health.

It's important to figure out who your friends are and which ones have your best interests at heart. So often we give people who are not our friends the power to hurt or discourage us. In the past few years, I've discovered that some people I thought were my friends turned out not to be. Others I considered just acquaintances turned out to be more than that. Some other people who didn't know I was alive a few years ago now think they're my bosom buddies, even though they're not. And I have another group who were my friends before I turned my life around, and they're still my friends now.

There's a spot in your life for all of them. But you may want to limit your time with people who don't share your goals, or whose negative attitudes might rub off on you. At the same time, try your best not to ram your philosophy down anyone's throat. Let your life be your most compelling argument—the glow of your complexion, the energy in each step you take. Either they'll get it—or they won't.

Dealing with Tough Situations

Please don't fool yourself by saying, "Well, she's stronger than I am" or, "I'll never be as good at all this as JoAnna."

I still have difficult spells, even after all these years. Just before that time of the month, when most women find themselves craving something sweet, I might succumb to a yearning for chocolate. But it'll be an extra piece of Healthy Exchanges Mexican Cinnamon Mocha Cake (page 272) instead of something high fat and unhealthy.

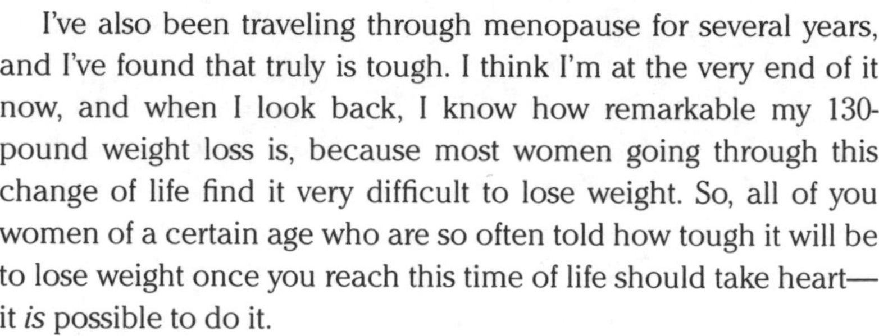

I've also been traveling through menopause for several years, and I've found that truly is tough. I think I'm at the very end of it now, and when I look back, I know how remarkable my 130-pound weight loss is, because most women going through this change of life find it very difficult to lose weight. So, all of you women of a certain age who are so often told how tough it will be to lose weight once you reach this time of life should take heart—it *is* possible to do it.

I've learned to cope so much better with difficult situations that in the past led me to "medicate" or numb myself with food. I finally realized that what was eating at me lots of times wasn't hunger but stress and emotional overload. Instead of dealing with the problem or the emotions, I ate.

Handling Anger

Now that I've learned to make sense of what was happening, to connect the two in my mind, it's not so likely that anger will act as an eating trigger. I've always been a pretty easygoing person, but if someone did something that upset me badly, instead of confronting them, I tended to clam up—and stuff food down my throat *to keep the anger in*.

Now I understand that, and I speak my mind much more.

Cliff told me he's noticed a tremendous difference in me, that I'm no longer meek, quiet, and subservient. I've learned to stand up for myself and speak my own mind. I'm not going to compromise any longer when it comes to what's important to me.

These days if I'm angry, instead of hanging up the phone and running toward the refrigerator, I let myself feel the anger, but I focus it on the person or situation instead of taking it out on myself. Sometimes I handle the frustration or fury by taking a walk or riding my bike, or else I go do something I enjoy. Other times, I'll sit down at the computer and start venting my emotions in my writing. (In fact, I think that's been the secret of the newsletter. While it was originally created to help other people and share what I've learned, it's also provided a real cleansing process for me.) As I sit at the computer, I usually come to terms with whatever has been bothering me.

I remember one particular newsletter that reached so deeply inside me, I cried for hours. What I'd written brought up to the surface emotions and fears I'd felt for years. Now I'd finally connected and understood what it was, and I figured out how I could share what I'd learned with others.

Sharing my innermost feelings and thoughts—that was the hardest thing to do from the beginning. It took me about three issues to get to the point where I could share the details of my personal struggle. I kept thinking, What are other people going to think? What will my family say? When instead of thinking less of me, they supported all I did, I began sharing more and more.

Writing about my journey to leading a healthy life, about losing weight and finding my work, really became a healing process for me. Maybe keeping a personal diary of your own journey will help you heal some old hurts, too.

What do you do with all those emotions? I liken it to what I went through when I obtained an annulment from my first marriage. Having to answer all those questions was so emotionally draining. But at the end of the process, I had worked through my anger and resentment toward my ex-husband, and I was left with just true sorrow that things hadn't turned out as I'd hoped they would when I said "I do." The pain subsided, and I was ready to move on.

Anyone can give up. It takes daily doing to keep up!

—Anonymous

Coping with Setbacks

One result of this process has been learning to handle the setbacks that are part of every life. Again, I'm never going to be Saint JoAnna. But that doesn't mean that when I have a bad day I can say, "Aw, heck," and go back to the way things were.

For a long time, I used to give myself permission not to walk on rainy days, even though I knew I'd feel better if I exercised. Now, I walk in the house or go to the Hart Center to walk. At least, I usually do. But I have days when I say it's just not worth it to eat healthily or make time for exercise. I tell myself I'm too busy, I'm tired, or I didn't sleep well. Pretty soon, though, I make a deal with myself. I say, "Look, I do feel better when I move, and I do feel better when I eat healthily, and when I just do what I'm supposed to be doing."

If you make up your mind you can't do something, you're absolutely right.

I tell myself, "Do it for just five minutes, and if you don't want to keep doing it, you can stop." Of course, just about every time I do keep going and making my healthy choices.

I use the same technique when I'm working. If a recipe I'm trying out fizzles or disappoints me in some way, I remind myself it's part of the experimental process. I learn from it, analyze what happened, file it in the back of my brain, and let my subconscious work on the problem. Then I go and try something else. Before I know it, I usually have it figured out.

It's very common—and much too easy—to get into a rut, especially after years of dieting. Boredom is one of the reasons people go off their diets, so it's important not to let yourself fall into that trap. You have to add variety, keep changing things. It's great to enjoy your favorite dishes, but at least once a week, *try something new*. If you always make linguine, buy some pasta shells or rotini. If you think you don't like Mexican food, give one of my South-of-the-Border recipes a try. Boredom and monotony are the first steps on the path toward falling off the wagon.

A lot of people like the idea of always knowing what they're supposed to eat, and they feel *safe* eating the same things day after day. Well, life isn't meant to be totally safe. If that were the case, we'd never leave our houses and we'd never do anything. Part of healthy living is really enjoying every part of your life. I've had my fill of that "safe" diet food—and I'll never do it again.

What did I have to show for it, except 56-inch hips?

Let's put those old tapes to rest once and for all. Repeat after me: I will never be perfect. I may never be skinny. But I no longer draw my self-esteem from my waist and hip measurements.

When you finally believe that you are worth loving, slender or heavy, young or older, and you love yourself before loving others, you'll find you can cope with anything life tosses your way.

When Others Make You Doubt Yourself

Taking pride in my accomplishments, discovering I had the strength to handle the rough spots, has been another important way my life has been changed for the better by following the HELP way of life.

A few years ago now, but still as fresh as ever in my memory, a former co-worker came over to my desk on my last day at work. By then I'd lost 125 pounds and gotten to the point where I'd decided to leave my insurance career to work full-time on Healthy Exchanges. This woman sat down and said to me, "JoAnna, what are you going to do when you gain back all the weight and you don't have a job to come back to?"

It was a true slap in the face, and it fed the fears that burned within me. It also hurt to have someone I'd worked with for years show so little faith.

But it was also a wake-up call. I knew that if I ever started to treat this as a diet, I would probably have to face that question—and I was more determined than ever not to.

Her question told me that some people might be waiting for that to happen, waiting for me to fail. I don't think I'd expected that, but instead of crying or running from the room, I was ready to handle it. I took a deep breath and faced her down. I said, "Well, I'm just not going to let that happen." Because I'd learned how to deal with difficult emotions during the past couple of years, I could deal with the bad feelings without resorting to a binge.

For so many years, I'd felt bad when I heard nasty remarks about my being overweight. Now I'd come such a long way, accomplished so much, and yet there were still people whose comments could hurt me. Around the same time as the first encounter, another co-worker said (in a remark that was repeated to me by another "friend"), "Well, she's no Skinny Minnie. Who does she think she is, telling other people how to lose weight?"

Ouch. Again, her comments tapped right into my fears, those pockets of doubt that still lived inside me. My first reaction was, Maybe she's right, maybe I shouldn't be telling people what to do. But then I said to myself, "JoAnna, you haven't come this far in building up your self-esteem to let someone else maliciously tear it down."

When someone says something mean or jealous like that, it still hurts. But I can't control the actions or words of other people. Nine out of ten people I know couldn't be happier for me about my weight loss and the success of Healthy Exchanges. I can't worry about pleasing everyone or persuade someone who feels bitter or jealous toward me to change. I think Rick Nelson said it best: "You can't please everyone, so you gotta please yourself."

How can you protect yourself from what people might say? Try to remember that it's their problem, not yours. In my case, I reminded myself I had hard evidence that I *knew* what I was talking about. I've got the letters and audiences to prove it. I've also got the old size-28 slacks I proudly show when speaking in public!

There are times when I've been tempted to just give up, but I realize that the healthier lifestyle I've now adopted has been a positive reinforcement for me to keep on going. Maybe I will get back to my goal weight; maybe I'll just stay where I am. In either case, it's a lot better than where I was.

I try not to be too hard on myself and realize I may have been too strict before. I will never fit into that 100 percent perfect mold, but that's all right.

—M. D., IA

Acceptance at Last

I can't tell you how many people have said to me, "I wish I were the weight I was when I first thought I was fat."

But that's the past, and you can't change it. I tell people that they have to accept themselves *now* and realize that time marches on. Maybe they'll never see that skinny size again. If they'll do *anything* to be that size again, they probably won't be able to sustain it. But if they lose weight to feel better for the rest of their lives, I believe they'll lose it and keep it off for good.

Sometimes, though, I have trouble listening to and believing what I've said to others. Even though I've accepted myself for who I am and what I am, I heard those whispering doubts in my mind again before I went to New York to meet with book publishers.

Why? Because when I think of the diet industry, I know that most spokespersons are super-slender, usually sizes 2, 4, or 6. I was concerned that the people I'd be meeting couldn't accept a normal-sized person, a real person who'd lost a lot of weight in a healthy way but wasn't *thin*.

When I mentioned this at one of the meetings, people seemed surprised that I had been worried about this. On the contrary, they were impressed with my accomplishments and felt that my story would give other "real" people out there encouragement and hope.

What a weight off my shoulders! I'd made the mistake of assuming what someone else's opinion would be, and I was happy to be wrong. It was a good reminder that we sometimes get caught in trying to be what other people expect us to be, instead of what we want for ourselves.

It's particularly important to keep this in mind when determining a weight-loss goal. If I believed that the insurance company weight charts were absolutely right, I might still be struggling to lose another fifteen or twenty pounds—to fit into *someone else's idea* of perfect.

I'm not.

I'd like to lose another few pounds in the next few years, but I'm not trying to hit a particular number. I know it may seem hard to believe that, but it's true. I'm not haunted anymore by a number that will tell me I've made it at last, that I'm *perfect*.

But what about when you're starting out? Are you better off without a specific number as a goal? I think so. I believe it's best not to start with an exact number in mind, because it too easily becomes the central focus of your efforts.

When I began, my goal was to recapture my health, not to hit a particular weight. Once I started losing weight, I wanted to *continue* losing weight. At some point along the way I did start aiming for a specific weight goal—a figure that is fifteen pounds less than I weigh now.

As you get closer and closer to what *your body's* goal is, you can start fine-tuning your destination. That's what I did. When the weight begins to come off much more slowly, when you feel yourself losing energy or resistance, that's a sign you may be pushing past the point where your body feels at its optimum health.

Most national weight-loss support groups give you a goal that someone else has set for anyone and everyone of your height. That's the only criterion they use. Well, now you're going to let *your body* set your goal.

Are you afraid you won't be able to tell when you're getting near your goal? Don't be. You'll know by the way your body feels and looks that you're nearing your destination.

I'm not going to try for a size 10. If I did, I'd end up like a wrinkled prune in the process. I don't want the body of a teenager and the face of a senior citizen. I won't let someone else set my weight goal or determine my dress size. It's no one's business what anyone's weight goal or dress size is, anyway. It's important not to give a particular number psychological power over you.

If it's to be . . . it's up to me!

—B. W., CA

What Keeps You Motivated?

Each of us is motivated by different kinds of reminders. Some people like to tape a "fat" picture on the refrigerator as the ultimate motivator. I'm one of those who'd rather look at a picture of me at my best—or photos of my grandchildren.

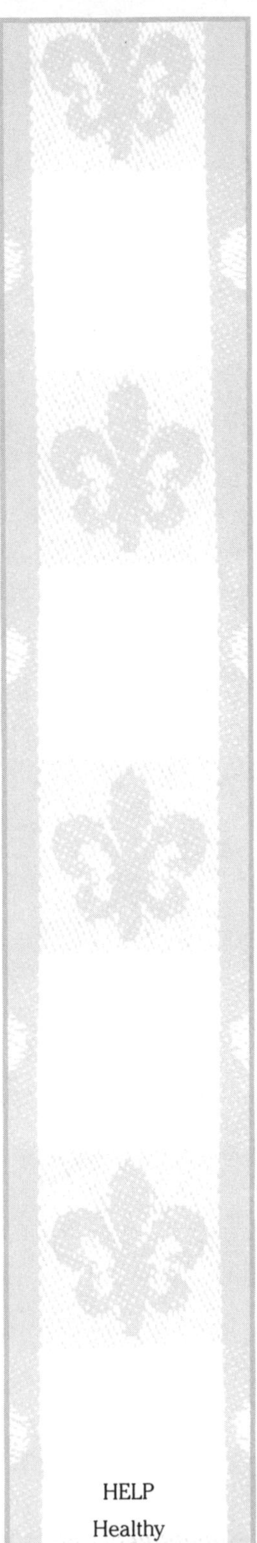

A lot of overweight people find a way not to be in pictures. Or they duck behind other people to hide their weight. When I saw a picture of me in a striped outfit at my highest weight, I wanted to destroy it. I didn't, though—I just hid it away. Then, when I had lost 100 pounds and was first sharing my cookbook, my son James said to me, "You know, Mom, you really need to show people where you've been, so they can see how far you've come." He remembered the picture of me in that striped outfit, and he said I should show it to people.

Part of me said no, never.

Part of me said, maybe—if it'll help someone else.

So I dug it out, but all the way down to the TV station where I was going to be interviewed, I didn't know whether or not I would show it. I finally said yes. When it flashed on the screen, I cringed in embarrassment. I thought people would laugh at it.

When that didn't happen, it became easier to share the picture, and now I show it everywhere I go. There are times when I look at it now, I can hardly believe that it's me, but it is. Healthy Exchanges and HELP made all the difference.

People ask me sometimes if I've had plastic surgery. I tell them, no, I haven't. Then they ask, "Well, how come your skin's so firm?" I answer that it's because I lost the weight slowly—slowly enough to be healthy, fast enough to see results. It's also because I eat healthy food, I exercise, I drink lots and lots of water every day (always have!), I've never been a sun worshiper, never smoked or drank, never caroused around—*and* I inherited good genes from my parents.

I don't think I'll ever have plastic surgery. I may sound like a broken record on this subject, but I believe it's best to accept yourself, be good to yourself, and be the person you are.

Losing Focus Once a Goal Is Reached

For many of us, reaching a big interim goal can produce a real feeling of psychological defeat instead of celebration. This is particularly true when we've rushed at a number on the scale by dieting strenuously and not making real lifestyle changes.

When I lost a lot of weight for my daughter Becky's wedding, it felt like finishing a race. When the wedding was over, I was at my most vulnerable—and I reverted to old eating behaviors right away. Usually, when you reach a weight-loss goal just for a special event, it's not sustainable for life.

Remember when Oprah Winfrey lost sixty-seven pounds on a liquid diet and rolled the wagonful of fat onto the stage? Then, her goal was just to get the weight off—at any cost, and with no clear plan about how to keep it off for the rest of her life. Before long, the weight came back. Only by changing her goals and methods has she finally gotten a real chance to sustain her success. This time, she's approached it as a *lifestyle change*, not a diet.

Many of us look at actors and athletes, at talk-show hosts with private chefs and trainers, and recognize that we can't duplicate their efforts, that often their goals aren't realistic for our lives. But we *can* make the choice to eat healthily, exercise moderately, and change our lives for keeps.

No More "On or Off"?

What's most important, and what can really make the difference between long-term success and heartbreaking failure, is to stop thinking about going *on* a diet or program. Going *on* means that we're thinking about sometime going *off*, that the way we're living has a time limit. Haven't you told yourself before that if you can just "behave" for three months, or six months, or a year, then you'll be able to go back to doing what you did before?

It's not true.

The changes we're talking about, the struggle we're in together, requires that we recognize we have to live in a healthy way for the rest of our lives. Someone sent me a quote for my Positive Attitude column that sums up this philosophy: "If you always do what you've always done, you'll always get what you always got." Simply put, if you go back to eating the way you did when you were overweight, if you go back to leading a totally sedentary lifestyle, you'll be back where you started—or even further away from your dream of better health.

This is not to say you'll never eat a hot-fudge sundae again, or have to skip the cake at your golden anniversary party. Heck, even Oprah confessed to downing three glasses of wine on Valentine's Day! But the next morning she went to the gym and exercised as

usual, and she ate three healthy meals that day. She got on with her life by recognizing that lapses happen, that we're human—but not helpless.

Let HELP Get You Over the Rough Spots

I think of HELP and Healthy Exchanges as more than a plan or a program. For me, it's a *way of life.* It's a little like raising children. You give them parameters, basic rules, but within those, they've got lots of freedom.

When you're struggling with a plateau or through trying times, remind yourself how the parts of HELP can make it easier on you and those you love.

Healthy Exchanges eating will give you the variety you crave and the real food you and your family can eat for a lifetime, not just until you've dropped a few pounds. The recipes are healthy and good tasting, prepared in reasonable portions, not tiny diet-size bites.

The moderate exercise I've suggested as part of HELP is a prescription for the rest of your life, echoed by doctors everywhere who recommend it to keep your heart healthy.

When you listen to your heart, you'll learn what dreams and goals still burn inside you, and by giving them a voice at last, you'll begin the journey of a lifetime to reach your heart's desires.

Finally, while you're struggling through any trying time, remember to give yourself credit for what you've already accomplished. You've done something positive for yourself for weeks or months, and *you deserve all the credit.*

You know how I keep saying, "Get on with life"? There's no better time to remember that than when the scale seems stuck, or the going gets tough. There's a whole world of people, places, and experiences out there. Get *off* the scale, get *out* of the house, and go meet all of it head-on!

Ten

Letting Go—and Moving On

Learn from yesterday . . .
Live for today . . .
Dream for tomorrow!

—B. W., IA

Sometimes it's easy to see what we want to "divest" from our lives—excess pounds or flabby thighs, for instance. Well, the previous chapters have given you all the tools and ideas you'll need to accomplish those kinds of goals.

But now I'd like to talk about some of the self-imposed and often hidden obstacles to success—hindrances we need to identify and let go of before we can fully follow the HELP lifestyle. Some of these include those favorite foods from childhood that may no longer be good for us, or those closetsful of clothing in a variety of sizes that we are hanging on to "just in case."

I believe we have to let go before we can move forward. "Letting go" of dieting was the way I began living healthily, but it was only the beginning.

Just as we feel a physical sense of liberation as the pounds begin to drop off, there is a similar sensation of freedom when we toss away old, unhealthy habits and comfort foods. For me, it was

donuts and hot-fudge sundaes (my all-time favorite binges when I tumbled off the Health Wagon) that I first had to give up. It wasn't nearly as hard as I expected. Because I enjoyed healthy desserts every day, the power these high-fat foods held over me quickly ebbed.

But, even as the pounds fell off, I learned that I had more housecleaning to do to get rid of my "excess baggage." And I'm still letting go as I continue to travel along the path to good health.

Letting Go of My "Fat" Clothes . . . and More

Every person who's ever lost and gained weight a dozen times knows what it's like to go down a couple of sizes and have to buy a new wardrobe. The smaller-size clothes fit for a few weeks or even months, then gradually they are relegated to the back of the closet as the old, larger-size clothes are regretfully pulled out and worn once more.

My closets were packed so tightly with clothes ranging from size 10 to size 28 that I could hardly get anything more into them! In the past, when I'd managed to starve myself down to a size 16 or 18, I just couldn't force myself to weed out the bigger clothes, because I knew that sooner or later I'd be wearing them again. And I refused to get rid of the size 10s I wore twenty years ago.

But one day I realized that all those closets full of clothing that didn't fit me anymore were a Catch-22. If I kept the clothes that were too large for me, I would never get rid of the safety net they represented. So, as the pounds started coming off, I gathered up all the oversized clothes and donated them to our local Goodwill. (There's nothing worse than being overweight and poor—your clothing selections are next to none. I always loved to design and sew my own clothing. I used to do with fabric what I now do with food. No matter what size I was, I had tons of clothes. Now I wanted someone else who needed attractive clothing in larger sizes to find what she needed.)

One time Cliff transported an entire pickup load to the shop. When he dropped the bags off, he told the workers, "I don't know how many clothes she has left at home, but if she ever gains the weight back again, she'll have to go stark naked!"

Letting go of large-size clothes is a strong statement that you're not going back up the scale. I remember a *People* magazine article that described how Oprah Winfrey was selling her large-size clothes (she has hundreds of outfits, and pricey ones!) and donating the money to charity. For her, too, letting go of her old wardrobe is a symbol that she isn't going back but moving forward—and full speed ahead!

After I set realistic goals for myself, I also realized I wasn't going to wear those size 10s ever again. Accepting that a size 12 or 14 was *who I was* helped me empty my closets of even more. It also helped me let go of those unrealistic expectations and get on with living my healthy lifestyle.

Letting Go of Childhood Trigger Foods

What else stood in my way? Like many people who've struggled with their weight, I needed to let go of certain trigger foods that brought back good memories from the past. We all have cozy feelings about certain foods, foods that help us relive pleasant times. But sometimes in order to move on, we have to separate the memory from the food. We can still enjoy remembering, but learn to let go of the unhealthy food.

Mine was butter. When I was growing up in the early fifties, my father worked in a local factory. Because the work was seasonal, Daddy was often laid off or on strike on my birthday. Back then, if you didn't work, you didn't get paid, so money was usually short when my birthday arrived.

Well, I loved the flavor of butter so much that all I wanted for my sixth birthday was a pound of real butter. Somehow my father scraped together the money to buy it, and my family celebrated with me (and that butter) at my birthday party supper. For the next twenty years, I ate anything I could spread with butter—I think I would have eaten wallpaper if it had been smeared with the creamy stuff!

Then, when I was in my late twenties, they told us butter was bad for us, so I switched to a margarine that said it contained no cholesterol. The brand I chose tasted almost as good as butter, so I kept on eating it—about two or three tubs of the stuff a week. No one bothered to tell me that it was still 100 percent fat!

When I started down the path to good health and began to

That which my mind can conceive,
And I dare to believe,
With God's help I can achieve.

look at the person I had become and still wanted to grow into, it finally clicked in my mind. All those years, I wasn't eating butter, I was trying to relive my fond memories of that birthday celebration. Once I made the connection, I could enjoy the memories, but without eating the excess fat. *I let it go.* Now I buy a single tub of reduced-calorie margarine, and it lasts me at least three months. I don't need that butter anymore. (In fact, when I see a big glob of it used on a cooking show or something, it actually turns my stomach!)

If you find you have an unnatural attachment to a particular food, something you really eat to excess, think about your childhood and try to figure out what it is about that food that makes you feel you have to have it. Think about the cozy memories the product gives you, just as that butter did me. I'll bet that you, too, can separate the memories from the food, cherish the memories, and get on with living in a healthy way.

Sometimes it's not a tough decision to give up an unhealthy food. A good friend, for example, gave up regular Pepsi without much difficulty. But other times there's more going on than just a taste for too much sugar. One of my subscribers wrote to me that she always let her kids have as much soda pop as they wanted, because she'd never been allowed to have it as a child. By letting them enjoy the sugary treats, she's still rebelling against her parents, but once she works that out in her own mind, I think she'll feel better about offering her children healthier drinks.

Letting Go of Old Hurt

I think the toughest part of letting go may be coming to terms with hurt feelings and finding a way to remove their power over us. Putting the past behind you may turn out to be a lifelong struggle, but I've found that it's only by facing the memories that still hurt me that I can truly move on.

I was haunted for years by recalling a party I went to when I was a plump young bride. There was this chair in the living room that no one was sitting on, so I walked over and sat down on it—and it started to creak and fall apart. This skinny girl laughed at me and said, "We were just waiting for someone like you to come in and sit on that chair." I felt so bad, I wanted to cry. I wanted to go home and disappear off the face of the earth. But I couldn't, because my husband was still enjoying the party.

I tried to get out of that room as fast as I could, but the pain of that encounter stayed with me for years. Life is really an equalizer, I discovered, because ten years later, that same woman was fighting her own weight problem. I often wondered if she remembered what she'd said to me, and if she'd had any idea how hurtful and cutting her remark was.

Most overweight people have stories just like that one, memories that still have the power to wound them to the heart even many years later. One that is still hard for me to think about involved someone I truly believed was my friend. We were at a business meeting, she'd had a few too many drinks, and she didn't know that I was nearby. She was joking about me to someone she'd just met, saying that I was at least a three-hundred-pound tubby. I was shattered. I couldn't believe that someone I considered a close friend could say such a thing about me. You know what I did the next day? I drowned my pain and anger in donuts. Did me a lot of good, right?

Remembering can hurt, but make peace with these memories, memories that tap into the fears you may always carry about regaining your weight. You'll get better at dealing with them. The longer you do it, the better you'll get. The goal is to diminish the power those memories have over you. You may always remember the hurt, but they can't rule you anymore.

I held the hurt of my "friend's" betrayal inside me for a long time, but finally I told Cliff how I felt, and he helped me get it out in the air. Sometimes it helps to share the pain with someone you trust, someone who will remind you that a true friend would never betray you like that. You have a right to expect your friends to defend you, not cut you down in front of others.

For a long time after that episode, whenever I thought about it, I wanted to reach for food for comfort. *I don't do that anymore.* At the same time I allow myself to remember the hurt, I've learned to let go of my instinctive reaction to it, which was to comfort myself with food. Even if it seems very difficult at first, eventually you'll get better at feeling the feelings and going on. It's necessary to acknowledge these feelings in order to start your own process of healing.

Do your best. Angels can do no better.

—V. B., IA

Letting Go of Friends Who Sabotage Us

Occasionally we have to let go of people who really are not our friends but what I call "friendly saboteurs." They're happiest when you're not eating healthily, either because they want a partner in crime or because it makes them feel superior when they're trim and you're not. If you have friends who are sabotaging your good efforts, *ask for their help*. If they truly care for you and want what's best for you, they'll gladly support you on your path to good health. If they continue to distract you from the path you've chosen, then it's up to you to decide whether it's time to let go of the friendship.

Then there are the people who watch every morsel that goes into your mouth. Don't you just want to scream when they ask, "Are you supposed to be eating that?" If someone shadows you on a regular basis, watching and waiting for you to slip or fail, they really aren't acting as friends do. Maybe you could thank them for being *so* interested in your healthy eating plan, but tell them firmly that the food that goes into your mouth is your business, and no one else's.

Sometimes old habits get in the way of your goal of living a healthy life. Are you still buying junk food because it's always been on your shopping list, or because "it's for the kids"? Do you still jump in the car to run an errand only three or four blocks away, instead of walking there? Do you clean off the plates after each meal by putting the extra food into your mouth instead of into the garbage so it "doesn't go to waste"? I could go on, but you get the idea.

I know change is hard. Sometimes it's really hard, and it takes a few tries to rid ourselves of a long-held behavior. But the more we let go and lighten our load, the easier it is to jump on the Health Wagon and ride it for the rest of our lives. Letting go is really the *only* way to go!

You Can Do It!

He who wants milk should not sit on a stool in the middle of a field expecting a cow to back up to him.

You've embarked on a journey that I hope you will find as satisfying and rewarding as I have. You've come such a long way already (did you realize that?) and you've learned so much about yourself, you're ready to enjoy the rest of your life.

After years of struggling to make your peace with food, you know now that you can live well in a world of sweet treats and eating on the run. Instead of fearing what havoc food may wreak on your life, you've grown to understand what a wonderful part of a healthy life good food can be.

You're breathing easier, too. By making walking, biking, swimming, and dancing a regular part of your life, you've filled your lungs with oxygen and your body with a new energy you may never have dreamed possible. You're becoming the person you were meant to be—with a glow on your cheeks, a sparkle in your eyes, and a heart that beats in time to the rhythm of life.

The future now belongs to you in a way it never did before. You've given a name to your hopes and dreams and made a promise to yourself that you will persevere toward those private, personal goals that make you feel prouder of yourself than you ever have.

Best of all, you've learned to believe in yourself, in your power to accomplish whatever you choose. You're the first to pat yourself on the back, you're no longer hiding your light under a bushel—and you've given yourself the rare gift of finding the good in the daily miracles of life.

In short, you've HELPed yourself. You've found a world of meaning behind that simple word—and begun to transform your life forever.

Now it's time to send you on your way with an outlook brimming with hope and all the inspiration I can provide.

I truly believe that life is meant to be enjoyed each and every single day. By focusing on what we want most and doing the best we can to reach those dreams, everything else in our lives will fall into place.

What is the emotional result of treating yourself well, of eating healthy food that you can enjoy with your family? You'll feel so much better inside and outside. You can see when people are treating themselves well because their skin just glows and their eyes shine with pleasure. Who would give that up for a sack of cake donuts?

People often ask me if I've had any cake donuts since I started Healthy Exchanges. (Especially those who knew me well, and knew how much I loved them!) Well, I've given myself permission to have cake donuts or candy bars—*if* I want them. At the state fair last year, they were giving away donuts. It was late in the afternoon, so I said to myself, well, I *can* have this if I want to, and count it as a snack. It would have been an acceptable snack for me. I took one bite and threw the rest away. What on God's earth did I ever think was so tasty about those little balls of fat? As for candy bars, I haven't had one yet, but I do have a healthy piece of pie on a fairly regular basis, and maybe because I enjoy a satisfying dessert so often, I don't miss them.

I never let myself forget that for twenty-eight years, I dreaded the arrival of spring because it meant shedding my heavy winter coat that concealed those 56-inch hips. I kept hoping for a magical cure to my "end-of-wintertime blues." For twenty-eight years, I dreaded the arrival of the fall holiday season, because I knew I would gain at least ten pounds between Thanksgiving Day and New Year's Eve. Instead of welcoming the warm days of summer, instead of celebrating the meaning of Christmas and the joyful times with family and friends, I thought only of hiding my oversized body and struggling to resist all the goodies everywhere I looked.

But with HELP, and with hard work, I reclaimed the pleasures of each new season's arrival. I now look forward to each new day, each new experience, each new person I meet.

Do you feel as excited contemplating your new road as I feel on your behalf? I hope so. But before I let you go, I'd like to repeat one word to you: MODERATION. The word *moderation* has been the cornerstone of Healthy Exchanges since that day more than five years ago when I quit dieting and started living a healthy life.

The dictionary defines moderation as 1) freedom from excess; 2) proper restraint; and 3) calmness. That just about sums up how I live now. I don't starve, and I don't overeat. I don't lie around on the couch instead of exercising, but I'm not obsessed enough to think I have to do at least two hours of exercise each day. I don't dwell on what can't be changed, and I refuse to live in a dreamworld of what isn't real.

I'm free from the chains of dieting. I practice proper restraint in my enjoyment of good food (at least most of the time!). And I now have a calmness in my life that no diet pill or donut could ever provide.

If I could give you three short pieces of inspirational advice, they would be:

- Never give up on yourself.
- Take life one day at a time, do the best you can for today, and let tomorrow take care of itself.
- With God's help, all things are possible.

Say to yourself, "I can live healthily just for today. And as the 'just for todays' add up, I can do this for the rest of my life."

From the day I started sharing my healthy lifestyle, people began to share their dreams with me, dreams they wanted to make come true for themselves. Helping to make their dreams come true with my recipes and my HELP plan, I feel that I have been truly blessed.

Just the other day I got a letter that brought tears to my eyes. A woman wrote to me from West Virginia and said, "Thank you for being our 'Moses' and leading us out of the desert of despair of being overweight and unhealthy."

No, thank *you* for letting me know how much what I'm doing means to you. The journey to good health that we're sharing together means more to me than you will ever know. Now I can't envision a future when my two "C"s—computer and cookstove—are not central to my existence. I plan on writing my newsletter and sharing a cookbook a year for the rest of my life—until I go to cookbook heaven, and then I hope to specialize in angel food cake!

How is all this possible? I am walking testimony to my belief that:

Prayer without work is doomed to failure.
Work without prayer won't be sustained long-term.
But—prayer combined with work creates miracles!

The next time you think that you just can't "do it," whatever your "do it" is, think of me. If a fifty-year-old woman, living in the middle of the cornfields in Iowa, who'd been a diet failure for twenty-eight years, who'd never written a single word for the public eye in forty-seven years, who had never spoken in front of an audience, let alone shared some very private sins, and who didn't even like to cook before stirring up Healthy Exchanges recipes, can "do it," can achieve what I have, then I know you have it within your power to "do it," too.

You may have noticed I like to share inspirational phrases that keep me going through the trying times. Here's one I came up with that truly sums up everything I believe in:

Dream your dreams,
Work your work,
Pray your prayers—
And your dreams, too, will come true.

If I did it, YOU CAN TOO!

Part Four

The Menus and Recipes

Eleven

Creating Healthy Exchanges Menus

Throughout this book, I've shared my philosophy that eating the Healthy Exchanges way means taking pleasure in what you eat, after years when eating meant either being deprived (and following a restrictive diet) or feeling guilty about eating "normal" food.

I've promised you it's possible to eat healthy, appetizing meals and enjoy every bite, and now I'm going to show you how to do it—with quick, easy, and mouthwatering dishes you can choose to prepare any day of the week. These are low-fat, low-sugar, yet high-flavor "common folk" recipes that everyone in your family will savor—and even ask for seconds! I think you may be surprised at just how good tasting and surprisingly like "real-people" food they are.

Before I outline the menus I've planned for your Healthy Exchanges sample week, let me repeat something I said earlier: You won't hurt my feelings if you don't follow my week's worth of menus *exactly.* This isn't about eating what *I* like, but about what *you* enjoy. We all have different tastes, different schedules, and different ideas about what foods give us pleasure. I want you to consider the following menus as suggestions and adjust them to please yourself.

You'll see—and maybe feel a bit overwhelmed—that *every* part of *every* meal is prepared from a Healthy Exchanges recipe. I did that on purpose, to show you all the different ways you can use Healthy Exchanges, *if you choose to.* But I don't expect you to do it all the time—so neither should you!

I've received lots of mail telling me that these recipes are surefire winners, so I'm confident you'll feel the same way about them. You've got a delicious journey ahead of you, one that will tickle your taste buds and show you just how good healthy food can be!

How Healthy Exchanges Menus Measure Up

If I tried to paint you a picture showing me eating an exact number of food choices, calories, fat grams, or exchanges *every single day,* it would be a *fake.* You should know by now that I LIVE IN THE REAL WORLD! Nothing in life comes out exactly—and so it is with what we choose to eat.

Some days, we're hungrier than others. We may dine out or celebrate with friends and choose to eat more of a particular food than we would at another time. Sometimes we feel stressed to the max—and need a little more healthy food to get us through.

These menus average out to about 1,600 calories a day. I've based the number of Weight Loss Choices, the approximately 20 percent of calories from fat, and the Diabetic Exchanges on this number. This is enough to keep your tummy filled and still allow you to lose weight slowly and surely. The actual calories will range from around 1,450 to 1,750, and the percentage of calories from fat will be as low as 15 percent on some days and as high as 25 percent on others. But the count for the week will average out to about 20 percent. (Remember, less than 15 percent is just another version of a diet—and more than 25 percent is too much of a good thing when eaten on a regular basis.)

In fact (if you care about such details!), the *actual daily averages* for the week are 1,619 calories and 35 grams of fat (or about 17 percent of calories coming from fat).

One last point about these measurements: The 1,600-calorie average is based on the needs of an average person with an average activity level. If you are middle-aged, inactive, or have a small build, you may not need so many calories. If you are young, very active, or have a large build, you may need more. So, adjust your daily needs accordingly. Also, if you have any medical problems or concerns, I want you to promise me you will seek sound medical advice *before* you start following this or any other food plan. This book is intended only as a guide, not as a substitute for medical advice.

Making the Menus Fit

No menu planner, especially mine, is written in stone. Always look the plan over and ask yourself, "Will this work for me and my family?" If parts of it won't, *change those parts so that they do.*

If you always eat brunch and dinner on Sundays instead of the three meals you enjoy on weekdays, the Healthy Exchanges Lifetime Plan provides the flexibility and freedom for you to continue doing so. You may decide to take some elements of my proposed breakfast and lunch on that day and include them in your family brunch. Or—you may completely redraft the menu to suit your food preferences, what's fresh in the market, even what you have left over in the freezer from a previous meal. *It's your choice.*

You may feel more confident choosing one or two dishes from each meal and incorporating those into a menu you plan yourself. You may be starting your healthy-living program in a week when you'll be eating several lunches out or having company for dinner. Maybe the weather is so great, you've decided to organize a picnic or a cookout.

Once you accept the philosophy of Healthy Exchanges eating and remind yourself that the primary goal is not to lose weight as fast as possible so you can get back to your old eating habits, you can use the information in this book to begin shaping a lifelong healthy-eating plan that fills you up, slims you down, and adds the benefits of good health to your life from now on.

Besides teaching you to prepare healthy recipes, I want to encourage you to take the time to develop a host of good habits . . . habits you can live with for the rest of your life.

How the Menus Work

I planned these menus around three healthy meals a day (plus two snacks), and I included *all* the recipes. I know it looks like a lot of work to prepare everything as laid out (it's less than you think!), but I wanted you to see all the possibilities and to give you some guidance in creating your own menus later on.

My goal here is to show you that you can enjoy foods you thought were "off-limits" as long as they are prepared in a healthy way. So—don't be surprised to find delicious desserts included every single day. I told you that was one of the reasons Healthy Exchanges has worked for me long-term, and I believe it will do the same for you.

I always make sure all the basic nutrition bases are covered each day before I add in the "extras." But I know how important those extras are to keeping you and your family from feeling deprived, and so I make sure they're a part of regular meals, not saved just for special occasions.

If you don't feel comfortable right away with this "common folk" healthy approach to eating, I'll understand. After all, it took me twenty-eight years before I finally saw the connection between permanent weight loss and enjoying healthy, attractive food in normal-sized portions. My satisfied tummy and my decreasing measurements convinced me at last that the closer the food was in flavor and appearance to the types of foods I grew up with, the better!

Look, if you're not satisfied by what you're eating, it won't matter how healthy it is. Before long, you'll be reaching for unhealthy foods to feed the hunger for taste and texture that still burns inside you—and you won't be developing lifelong healthy eating habits.

These Healthy Exchanges recipes will feed that hunger inside, whether you've been longing for creamy soups, spicy main dishes, or sweet treats to soothe your soul. Here's to a delicious new beginning!

Brown Bagging It the Healthy Exchanges Way

One of the daily challenges for most of us is figuring out what to bring for lunch to work or school, and how to keep from getting into an eating rut. One of the most popular columns in my monthly newsletter is "Brown Bagging It," in which I share some good ideas and offer recipes that are easy to transport, simple to heat up, and delicious to enjoy when you're dining away from your own kitchen table. Too many people with a history of dieting tend to "settle" for dull and boring when it comes to the contents of their lunch bags: cans of water-packed tuna, hard-boiled eggs, some carrot sticks—NO MORE!

It's time to change the way you think of your brown-bag lunch—especially since so many offices now provide refrigerators and microwaves. Your best purchase: a good wide-mouth thermos, so you can enjoy hearty soups and meaty chili in the colder months, or anytime at all. Most of my soup recipes can be prepared while you're getting dressed for work and packed to go in a couple of minutes. Accompanied by some crunchy fat-free crackers, the soup makes a satisfying meal. If you've got a sweet tooth, you can add a piece of Healthy Exchanges dessert instead of just an apple or orange (although I usually like fresh fruit for lunch—it leaves me feeling energetic and ready to handle the afternoon ahead!).

If you were raised to expect your big meal at midday, and you still miss sitting down to a multi-course menu then, it's all right to satisfy that longing by planning a lunch that includes several different dishes. (That's the way we eat at my house because I'm usually testing four or five different things at once!) Have a cup of healthy soup with a cracker, then perhaps a tasty carrot salad (filling and easy to fix). A stuffed pita, bagel, or sandwich is both a handy main course and a satisfying one; I like to use thin-sliced bread to give myself a two-slice sandwich for just one bread exchange. And don't forget dessert . . . any number of my recipes travel well.

Not bad for a brown-bag working lunch at your desk or on the run! The important thing to remember is, you don't need to suffer or give up the simple pleasure of a homemade packed lunch just because you've chosen to eat healthily. I bet you'll find that everyone in the lunchroom wants a taste, a piece, or even to trade lunches with you, because everything you're eating looks and tastes so good.

If you're an early riser, fixing your brown-bag lunch in the morning will work just fine. But if you're always racing out the door with your breakfast in your purse and your hair not quite dry, then take a few minutes before bed the night before and lay out the fixings for your lunch just as you lay out your clothes. It's important for you to feel good about how you look when you go to work, but it's also important to strengthen your commitment to healthy eating by banishing the excuse of "I didn't have time . . ."

So—enjoy your healthy lunch, share your secrets if anyone asks (it's the *kind* thing to do!), and try to leave five to fifteen minutes at the end of your lunch break for a walk. Besides being good for your heart, it'll help your digestion—and send you back to your desk feeling really good!

Sample Menus for One Week of Healthy Exchanges

Yes, I know—you usually start a new diet on a Monday . . . and find yourself falling off the wagon by Tuesday or Wednesday. Healthy Exchanges isn't a diet, so let's begin your new way of eating on a day when you can take time to eat with your family—or simply give yourself the gift of eating a satisfying meal on a day off from work.

Sunday

Breakfast

Lemon Pancakes with Blueberry Sauce with 1 cup skim milk	288

Lunch

Shrimp Caesar Salad	245
Frosted Orange Salad	241
Peach Melba Daiquiri	292

Dinner

French Onion Soup	232
or Iowa Corn Chowder	233
Frisco Salad	241
Molded Relish Salad	242
Creamy Mashed Potatoes	251
or Twice-Baked Potatoes with 2 teaspoons reduced-calorie margarine	254
Chicken Breasts with Raspberry Sauce	256
South Seas Chocolate Tarts	276

Snack

Paradise Yogurt	291

Snack

Wacky Spice Cake	277

Note: Coffee, tea, and diet beverages may be used *in moderation* as you choose. Try to drink at least eight glasses of water during the day.

Monday

Breakfast

Jo's Granola with 1 cup skim milk	288

Lunch

Tuna-Cheddar Sandwiches	264
or Tuna-Macaroni Stuffed Tomatoes	265
Italian Copper Pennies	253
or Cauliflower and Tomato au Gratin	250
Oatmeal Bars	273

Dinner

Onion Noodle Soup	235
or Italian Zucchini Tomato Soup	234
Mediterranean Tomatoes	253
Deviled Carrots	252
or Wimp's Fresh Salsa	254
Easy "Lasagna" Casserole	258
Raspberry Cream Tarts	275

Snack

Baked Apple	269

Snack

Party Mix	292
Banana Nog	280

Tuesday

Breakfast

Breakfast-in-Hand Sandwich with 1 cup skim milk	282

Lunch

Ranchero Vegetable Salad	244
Chili Kolaches	257
or Chicken Taco Salad	257
Frozen Yogurt Tarts	271

Dinner

Spinach Salad	246
French Carrot Salad	240
Fish Creole	259
or Easy Veggie-Ham Dish	259
Almost Sinless Sundae Pie	268

Snack

Strawberry Shake	294

Snack

Ham-Spinach Dip with Veggies	287
Taffy Apple Salad	246

Wednesday

Breakfast

Olé Scrambled Eggs
with 1 cup skim milk 290

Lunch

Lifesaver Soup 234
or Quick Chicken Soup 235
Waldorf Chicken Salad Pitas 265
S'Mores Pudding 275

Dinner

Deli Coleslaw 239
Green Bean Salad 242
Macaroni and Cheese with Tomatoes 262
or Grandma's Salmon Loaf 260
Dwayne's Coconut Banana Chocolate Cream Pie 271

Snack

Peanut Butter and Jelly Pizza Snack 293
or Cherry Kolaches 270

Snack

Candy Drops 282
Orange Jo 291

Thursday

Breakfast

Breakfast Bread Pudding 281
Mocha 290

Lunch

Fiesta Corn Salad 240
Old-Style Slaw 243
Italian Loose Meat Sandwiches 261
or Bubble Pizza 256
Dewy Mountain Strawberry Cheesecake 270
"Homemade" Limeade 287

Dinner

Cauliflower-Broccoli-Raisin Salad 238
or Tomato, Celery, and Cabbage Salad 247
Breezy Green Beans 250
Linguine with Tuna and Peas 261
Soda Fountain Delight 276

Snack

Fruity-Cheese Sandwich 286

Snack

Cheesy Popcorn with 1 cup skim milk 284

Friday

Breakfast

Cheese 'n' Fruit English with 1 cup skim milk 284

Lunch

Southwestern Vegetable Soup with 7 fat-free soda crackers 236

Cottage Cheese–Stuffed Tomatoes 239

New England Pumpkin Raisin Pie 274

Dinner

Chinese Egg Drop Soup 232

Blue Cheese Mushroom Salad 238

Polynesian Carrot Salad 243

Sweet 'n' Sour Pork 264

or Norwegian Burgers 263

Orange Pudding Treats 274

Snack

"Danish" Treat 285

Snack

Chocolate Chip Drop Cookies 285

Apple Orchard Lemonade 280

Saturday

Breakfast

Carrot-Raisin Muffin with 1½ teaspoons fat-free cream cheese and 1 tablespoon apple butter 283

Mexican Hot Chocolate 289

Lunch

Quick Spinach Salad 244

Hawaiian Chicken Salad 260

Lemon Rice Pudding 272

Dinner

Salsa Zucchini Salad 245

Grande Green Beans 252

or Corn-Zucchini Sauté 251

Mexican Scalloped Potatoes 262

Acapulco Gold Pudding 268

Snack

Blueberry "Ice Cream" 281

Snack

Grande Roma Dip 286

Potato Chips 293

Your Daily Menu Planner

Day: ______________________________

____

Breakfast: ______________________________

____

____

____

____

____

Lunch: ______________________________

____

____

____

____

____

Dinner: ______________________________

____

____

____

____

____

Snack(s): ______________________________

____

Twelve

Shopping the Healthy Exchanges Way

Sometimes, as part of a cooking demonstration, I take the group on a field trip to the nearest supermarket. There's no better place to share my discoveries about which healthy products taste best, which are best for you, and which ones don't deliver enough taste to include in my recipes.

While I'd certainly enjoy accompanying you to your neighborhood store, we'll have to settle for a field trip *on paper.* I've tasted and tried just about every fat- and sugar-free product on the market, but so many new ones keep coming all the time, you're going to have to learn to play detective on your own. I've turned label reading into an art, but often the label doesn't tell me everything I need to know.

Sometimes you'll find, as I have, that the product with *no* fat doesn't provide the taste satisfaction you require; other times, a no-fat or low-fat product just doesn't cook up the same way as the original product. And some foods, including even the leanest meats, can't eliminate *all* the fat. That's okay, though—a healthy diet should include anywhere from 15 to 25 percent of total calories from fat on any given day.

Take my word for it—your supermarket is filled with lots of delicious foods that can and should be part of your healthy diet for life. Come, join me as we check it out on the way to the checkout!

First stop, the **salad dressing** aisle. Salad dressing is usually a high-fat food, but there are great alternatives available. Let's look first at the regular Ranch dressing—2 tablespoons has 170 calories and 18 grams of fat—and who can eat just 2 tablespoons? Already, that's about half the fat grams most people should consume in a day. Of course, it's the most flavorful, too. Now let's look at the low-fat version. Two tablespoons have 110 calories and 11 grams of fat; they took about half of the fat out, but there's still a lot of sugar there. The fat-free version has 50 calories and zero grams of fat, but they also took most of the flavor out. Here's what you do to get it back: add a tablespoon of fat-free mayonnaise, a few more parsley flakes, and about a half teaspoon of sugar substitute to your 2-tablespoon serving. That trick, with the fat-free mayo and sugar substitute, will work with just about any fat-free dressing and give it more of that full-bodied flavor of the high-fat version. Be careful not to add too much sugar substitute—you don't want it to become sickeningly sweet.

I use Kraft fat-free **mayonnaise** at 10 calories per tablespoon to make scalloped potatoes, too. The Smart Beat brand is also a good one.

Before I buy anything at the store, I read the label carefully: the total fat plus the saturated fat; I look to see how many calories are in a realistic serving, and I say to myself, would I eat that much—or would I eat more? I look at the sodium and I look at the total carbohydrates. I like to check those ingredients because I'm cooking for diabetics and heart patients, too. And I check the total calories from fat.

Remember that 1 fat gram equals 9 calories, while 1 protein or 1 carbohydrate gram equals 4 calories.

A wonderful new product is I Can't Believe It's Not Butter spray, with zero calories and zero grams of fat in four squirts. It's great for your air-popped popcorn. As for **light margarine spread,** beware—most of the fat-free brands don't melt on toast, and they don't taste very good either, so I just leave them on the shelf. For the few times when I do use a light margarine I tend to buy Smart Beat Ultra, Promise Ultra, or Weight Watchers Light Ultra. The number-one ingredient in them is water, so they are not good choices for baked products. I occasionally use the light margarine in cooking, but I don't really put margarine on my toast anymore. I use apple butter or make a spread with fat-free cream cheese mixed with a little spreadable fruit instead.

So far, Pillsbury hasn't released a reduced-fat **crescent roll,** so I recommend only one crescent roll per serving. I usually make eight of the rolls serve twelve by using them for a crust. The house brands may be lower in fat, but they're usually not as good flavor-wise—and don't quite cover the pan when you use them to make a crust. If you're going to use crescent rolls with lots of other stuff on top, then a house brand might be fine.

The Pillsbury French Loaf makes a wonderful **pizza crust** that fills a giant jelly roll pan. One-fifth of this package "costs" you only 1 gram of fat (and I don't even let you have that much!). Once you use this for your pizza crust, you will never go back to anything else. I use it to make calzones, too.

I only use Philadelphia Fat-Free **cream cheese** because it has the best consistency. I've tried other brands, but I wasn't happy with them. Healthy Choice makes lots of great products, but their cream cheese just doesn't work as well with my recipes.

Let's move to the **cheese** aisle. My preferred brand is Kraft ⅓ Less Fat Shredded Cheeses. I will not use the fat-free versions because *they don't melt.* I would gladly give up sugar and fat, but I will not give up flavor. This is a happy compromise. I use the reduced-fat version, I use less, and I use it where your eyes "eat" it, on top of the recipe. So you walk away satisfied and with a finished product that's very low in fat. If you want to make grilled cheese sandwiches for your kids, use the Kraft ⅓ Less Fat cheese slices, and it'll taste exactly like the one they're used to. The fat-free kind will not.

Some brands have come out with a fat-free **hot dog,** but the ones we've tasted haven't been very good. So far, among the low-fat brands, I think Healthy Choice tastes the best. Did you know that regular hot dogs have as many as 15 grams of fat?

Dubuque's Extra-Lean Reduced-Sodium **ham** tastes wonderful, reduces the sodium as well as the fat, and gives you a larger serving. Don't be fooled by products called turkey ham; they may *not* be lower in fat than a very lean pork product. Here's one label as an example: I checked a brand of turkey ham called Genoa. It gives you a 2-ounce serving for 70 calories and 3½ grams of fat. The

Dubuque extra-lean ham, made from pork, gives you a 3-ounce serving for 90 calories, but only 2½ grams of fat. *You get more food and less fat.*

The same can be true for packaged **ground turkey;** if you're not buying *fresh* ground turkey, you may be getting a product with turkey skin and a lot of fat ground up in it. Look to be sure the package is labeled with the fat content; if it isn't, run the other way!

Your best bets in **snack foods** are pretzels, which are always low in fat, as well as the chips from the Guiltless Gourmet, which taste especially good with one of my dips.

Frozen dinners can be expensive and high in sodium, but it's smart to have two or three in the freezer as a backup when your best-laid plans go awry and you need to grab something on the run. It's not a good idea to rely on them too much, though—what if you can't get to the store to get them, or you're short on cash? The sodium can be high in some of them because they often replace fat with salt, so do read the labels. Also ask yourself if the serving size is enough to satisfy you; for many of us, it's not.

Egg substitute is expensive and probably not necessary unless you're cooking for someone who has to worry about every bit of cholesterol in his or her diet. If you occasionally have a fried egg or an omelet, *use the real egg.* For cooking, you can usually substitute two egg whites for one whole egg. Most of the time it won't make any difference, but check your recipe carefully.

Frozen pizzas aren't particularly healthy, but used occasionally, in moderation, they're okay. Your best bet is to make your own using the Pillsbury French Loaf. Take a look at the frozen pizza package of your choice, though, because you may find that plain cheese pizza, which you might think would be the healthiest, could actually have the most fat. Since there's nothing else on there, they have to cover the crust with a heavy layer of high-fat cheese. A veggie pizza generally uses less cheese and more healthy, crunchy vegetables.

Healthy frozen desserts are hard to find except for the Weight Watchers brands. But I've always felt that their portions are so small, and for their size still pretty high in fat and sugar. (This is one of the reasons I think I'll be successful marketing my frozen desserts someday. After Cliff tasted one of my earliest healthy pies—and licked the plate clean—he remarked that if I ever opened a restaurant, people would keep coming back for my desserts alone!) Keep an eye out for fat-free or very low-fat frozen yogurt or sorbet products. Even Häagen-Dazs, which makes some of the highest fat content ice cream, now has a fat-free fruit sorbet pop out that's pretty good. I'm sure there will be more before too long.

You have to be realistic: What are you willing to do, and what are you *not* willing to do? Let's take bread, for example. Some people just have to have the real thing—rye bread with caraway seeds or a whole-wheat version with bits of bran in it.

I prefer to use reduced-calorie **bread** because I like a *real* sandwich. This way, I can have two slices of bread and it counts as only one bread/starch exchange.

Do you love **croutons?** Forget the ones from the grocery store—they're extremely high in fat. Instead, take reduced-calorie bread, toast it, give it a quick spray of I Can't Believe It's Not Butter spray, and let it dry a bit. Cut the bread in cubes. Then, for an extra-good flavor, put the pieces in a plastic bag with a couple of tablespoons of Kraft fat-free Parmesan cheese and shake them up. You might be surprised at just how good they are! Another product that's really good for a crouton—Corn Chex cereal. Sprinkle a few Chex on top of your salad, and I think you'll be pleasantly surprised. I've also found that Rice Chex, crushed up, with parsley flakes and a little bit of Parmesan cheese, makes a great topping for casseroles that you used to put potato chips on.

Salad toppers can make a lot of difference in how content you feel after you've eaten. Some low-fat cheese, some homemade croutons, and even some bacon bits on top of your greens deliver an abundance of tasty satisfaction. I always use the real Hormel **bacon bits** instead of the imitation bacon-flavored bits. I only use a small amount, but you get that real bacon flavor—and less fat, too.

How I Shop for Myself

Shopping is almost like a social event with me. I stop and visit with people I might not otherwise see. I do make certain to bring my recipes with me so I can purchase all the ingredients I need. A lot of people tell me they just keep my cookbook or the latest newsletter in their purses. That way, they can quickly run in after work and pick up what they need. They like knowing it won't take more than a few minutes once they get home to put dinner on the table.

Most of the time I go to the store with a shopping list. I know what I need, and I shop for normal family needs usually once a week. I try to buy only enough to fit into two large bags so they can fit into the basket on my bike.

Of course, when I'm creating recipes, then I'll go to the store for any special ingredients I need. But often I make up recipes from what is already in my cupboard. Other times, because I'm preparing a meal as part of a presentation and may be serving as many as 100 people, I'll make a special visit to the store to get the ingredients I need.

I always keep my kitchen stocked with my basic staples; that way, I can go to the cupboard and create new recipes anytime I'm inspired. I hope you will take the time (and allot the money) to stock your cupboards with items from the staples list, so you can enjoy developing your own healthy versions of family favorites without making extra trips to the market.

I'm always on the lookout for new products sitting on the grocery shelf. When I spot something I haven't seen before, I'll usually grab it, glance at the front, then turn it around and read the label carefully. I call it looking at the promises (the "come-on" on the front of the package) and then at the warranty (the ingredients list and the label on the back).

If it looks as good on the back as it does on the front, I'll say okay and either create a recipe on the spot or take it home for when I do think of something to do with it. Picking up a new product is just about the only time I buy something not on my list.

The items on my shopping list are normal, everyday foods, but as low fat and low sugar *(while still tasting good)* as I can find. I can make any recipe in this book as long as these staples are on my shelves. After using these products for a couple of weeks, you will find it becomes routine to have them on hand. And I promise you, I really don't spend any more at the store now than I did a few years ago when I told myself I couldn't afford some of these items. Back then, of course, plenty of unhealthy, high-priced snacks I really didn't need somehow made the magic leap from the grocery shelves into my cart. Whom was I kidding?

Yes, you often have to pay a little more for fat-free or low-fat products, including meats. But since I frequently use a half pound of meat to serve four to six people, your cost per serving will be much lower.

Try adding up what you were spending before on chips and cookies, premium-brand ice cream and fatty cuts of meat, and you'll soon see that we've *streamlined* your shopping cart and taken the weight off your pocketbook as well as your hips!

Remember, your good health is *your* business—but it's big business, too. Write to the manufacturers of products you and your family enjoy but feel are just too high in fat, sugar, or sodium to be part of your new healthy lifestyle. Companies are spending millions of dollars to respond to consumers' concerns about food products, and I bet that in the next few years, you'll discover fat-free and low-fat versions of nearly every product piled high on your supermarket shelves!

Shopping List for Your Week of Menus

Don't be alarmed by the number of items you see in the lists below—you probably have many of these staples on your shelves already. If you're planning to make all eighty-five recipes this week, these are the ingredients you'll need, so plan to stock up on what you don't have.

If you're going to pick and choose among the recipes for your week's menus, then carefully check the list of ingredients in each recipe you select to make certain you have everything you will need. Life is definitely easier if you locate all the ingredients and place them on the counter before you start to cook. Many "recipe failures" have occurred because the cook didn't realize until it was too late that there wasn't any "whatever" in the refrigerator or cupboard. When the moment arrived to add that ingredient—disaster struck! Don't assume anything when it comes to necessary ingredients. A quart of milk that I'm certain I saw in the refrigerator just two hours earlier has a way of disappearing when my son is thirsty. I wouldn't be surprised if the same thing happens at your house.

Meat and Dairy

Reduced-calorie margarine
Eggs
Fat-free plain yogurt
Skim milk
Fat-free cottage cheese
Fat-free cream cheese
Shredded reduced-fat Cheddar cheese
Shredded reduced-fat mozzarella cheese
Grated American cheese
Kraft grated House Italian cheese
Chicken breasts
Extra-lean ground turkey or beef (at least 90% lean)
White fish fillets
Dubuque 97% fat-free ham
Lean pork tenderloins

Bread and Grains

Fat-free white bread
Reduced-calorie hamburger buns
Pita bread
Bisquick reduced-fat baking mix
English muffins
Popcorn
Reduced-sodium pretzels
Rice
Quick-cooking oats
Linguine
Noodles
Elbow macaroni
Rice Chex
Wheat Chex

Cheerios
Corn flakes

Fruits and Vegetables

Orange juice
Strawberries
Apples
Bananas
Raspberries
Lemons
Raisins
Potatoes
Onions
Cabbage
Iceberg lettuce
Romaine lettuce
Spinach
Prepackaged coleslaw mix
Celery
Carrots
Cauliflower
Broccoli
Mushrooms
Green bell peppers
Radishes
Green onions
Cilantro
Parsley
Cucumbers
Tomatoes

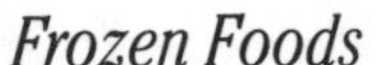

Frozen Foods

Green peas
Cut green beans
Cut carrots
Whole-kernel corn
Chopped spinach
Frozen shredded potatoes
Unsweetened strawberries
Blueberries
Yeast dinner rolls
Shrimp

Canned Goods

Healthy Request chicken broth
Beef broth
Healthy Request tomato soup
Healthy Request tomato juice
Reduced-calorie cranapple juice
Sliced mushrooms
Tomatoes
Hunt's chunky tomato sauce
Tomato sauce
Mexican stewed tomatoes
Chunky salsa
Crushed pineapple, packed in fruit juice
Pineapple chunks, packed in fruit juice
Mandarin oranges
Unsweetened applesauce
Pumpkin
French-style green beans
Pinto beans
Albacore tuna, packed in water
Evaporated skim milk

Spices and Condiments

Fat-free salad dressings: blue cheese, French, Catalina, Thousand Island, Ranch, Italian
Sprinkle Sweet or Sugar Twin
Equal
Brown Sugar Twin
Cinnamon
Apple pie spice
Pumpkin pie spice
Chili seasoning mix
White vinegar
Cider vinegar
Dried chives
Lemon pepper
Celery seed
Black pepper
Salt
Dried parsley flakes
Dried basil
Dried onion flakes
Coconut extract
Vanilla extract
Almond extract
Flour
Cornstarch
Baking soda
Baking powder
Unsweetened cocoa
Prepared mustard
Dijon mustard
Prepared horseradish
Pickle relish
Fat-free mayonnaise
Vegetable oil
Worcestershire sauce

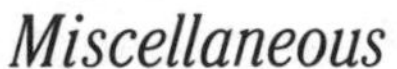

Miscellaneous

Sugar-free gelatin: orange, lemon, lime, strawberry, Hawaiian pineapple, cherry
Sugar-free instant pudding mix: vanilla, chocolate
Sugar-free Cook & Serve pudding mix: vanilla, chocolate
Nonfat dry milk powder
Swiss Miss sugar-free hot chocolate mix
Crystal Light lemonade mix
Crystal Light tropical punch mix
Diet 7UP
Diet Mountain Dew
Diet Coke
Lemon juice
Lime juice
Slivered almonds
Walnuts
Pecans
Spreadable fruit spread: raspberry, apricot, grape
Reduced-fat peanut butter
Apple butter
Cool Whip Lite
Fat-free and sugar-free vanilla "ice cream"
Maraschino cherries
Miniature chocolate chips
Miniature marshmallows
Keebler piecrusts: butter flavored, graham cracker, chocolate flavored
Keebler single-serve graham cracker pie shells
Cary's sugar-free maple syrup
Flaked coconut
Instant potato flakes
Bacon bits (real bacon, not imitation)
Fat-free corn chips
Cooking sprays: regular, butter flavored, olive oil flavored

A Peek into My Pantry and My Favorite Brands

Everyone asks me what foods I keep on hand and what brands I use. There are lots of good products on the grocery shelves today—many more than we dreamed about even a year or two ago. And I can't wait to see what's out there twelve months from now. The following are my staples and, where appropriate, my favorites *at this time.* I feel these products are healthier, tastier, easy to get—and deliver the most flavor for the least amount of fat, sugar, or calories. If you find others you like as well *or better,* please use them. This is only a guide to make your grocery shopping and cooking easier.

Fat-free plain yogurt (Yoplait)
Nonfat dry skim milk powder (Carnation)
Evaporated skim milk (Carnation)
Skim milk
Fat-free cottage cheese
Fat-free cream cheese (Philadelphia)
Fat-free mayonnaise (Kraft)
Fat-free salad dressings (Kraft)
Fat-free sour cream (Land O Lakes)
Reduced-calorie margarine (Weight Watchers, Smart Beat, *or* Promise)
Cooking spray:
  Butter flavored (Weight Watchers)
  Olive oil flavored and regular (Pam)
Vegetable oil (Puritan Canola Oil)
Reduced-calorie whipped topping (Cool Whip Lite *or* La Creme Lite)
Sugar substitute:
  if no heating is involved (Equal)
  if heating is required
   —*white* (Sprinkle Sweet *or* Sugar Twin)
   —*brown* (Brown Sugar Twin)

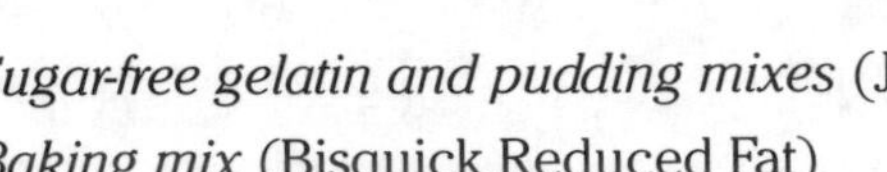

Sugar-free gelatin and pudding mixes (Jell-O)
Baking mix (Bisquick Reduced Fat)
Pancake mix (Hungry Jack Extra Lights *or* Aunt Jemima Lite)
Reduced-calorie syrup (Cary's Sugar-free Maple)
Parmesan cheese (Kraft's Fat-Free Topping *or* Kraft's Grated House Italian Cheese)
Reduced-fat cheese (Kraft, Healthy Favorites, *or* Weight Watchers)
Shredded frozen potatoes (Mr. Dell's)
Spreadable fruit (Smucker's, Welch's, *or* Sorrell Ridge)
Peanut butter (Peter Pan Reduced Fat, Jif Reduced Fat, *or* Skippy Reduced Fat)
Chicken broth (Campbell's Healthy Request)
Beef broth (Swanson)
Tomato sauce (Hunt's—Regular and Chunky)
Canned soups (Campbell's Healthy Request)
Tomato juice (Campbell's Healthy Request)
Ketchup (Campbell's Healthy Request *or* Heinz Lite)
Purchased piecrust:
unbaked (Pillsbury—from dairy case)
graham cracker, butter flavored, or chocolate flavored (Keebler)
90 percent lean pastrami or corned beef (Carl Buddig)
Luncheon meats (Healthy Choice)
97 percent fat-free reduced-sodium ham (Dubuque)
Lean frankfurters and Polish kielbasa sausage (Healthy Choice)
Canned white chicken, packed in water (Swanson)
90 percent lean ground turkey
90 percent lean ground beef
Canned tuna, packed in water (Starkist)
Soda crackers (Nabisco Fat-Free Premium)
Reduced-calorie bread—40 calories per slice or less (Colonial *or* Wonder Bread)
Hamburger buns—80 calories each (Colonial Old Fashioned)
Rice—instant, regular, brown, and wild

Instant potato flakes (Betty Crocker Potato Buds)
Noodles, spaghetti, and macaroni
Salsa (Chi Chi's Mild)
Pickle relish—dill, sweet, and hot dog
Mustard—Dijon, prepared, and spicy
Unsweetened apple juice
Unsweetened applesauce
Frozen fruit—no sugar added
Fresh fruit
Fresh, frozen, and canned vegetables
Spices
Lemon and lime juice
Instant fruit beverage mixes (Crystal Light)
Dry dairy beverage mixes (Nestlé's Quik, *and* Swiss Miss)
"Ice Cream" (Well's Blue Bunny Fat-Free *and* Sugar-Free Dairy Dessert, Weight Watchers)

If your grocer does not stock these items, why not ask if they can be ordered on a trial basis? If the store agrees to do so, be sure to tell your friends to stop by, so that sales are good enough to warrant restocking the new products. Competition for shelf space is fierce, so only products that sell well stay around.

Thirteen

How I Create Healthy Exchanges Recipes

Are you wondering how I come up with so many different healthy recipes month after month, year after year? I've only got a small galley kitchen, not some fancy test kitchen with acres of appliances. Well, aside from my family, the love of my life is creating and testing my "common folk" healthy recipes. I create about three hundred new recipes every month, and taste-test at least ninety to one hundred of them! I never leave home without paper, pens, and calculator, and I'm always jotting down ideas. (Cliff says he can almost see the smoke coming out of the pen!)

I can see, smell, taste, and feel the finished product in my mind before I ever begin writing. I take credit for chopping the onions and even for washing the dishes, but I won't take credit for the ideas that flow like water. I believe this is a gift from God meant to be shared with anyone who wants to cook in my "common folk" healthy way.

Now, where do all those recipe ideas come from? From just about anywhere you can imagine! I started by revising my family favorites, experimenting with ways to banish excess fats, sugars, and sodium while retaining the original flavor. (And I always made them easier to prepare in the process.)

When I discover new products in the grocery store, ideas for new recipes seem to boil over one right after the next. Once I check that the new item truly delivers the healthy food promised on the label, I start thinking of ways to use it.

I also eat food "with my eyes" when we dine out in restaurants. I read the menu for ideas, and if there's a display case or tray I look over the salads and desserts to see what looks good. I also look at food served to others (though I try not to stare!), and I've even been inspired to create a recipe by a mouthwatering billboard outside a restaurant.

I love to look at pictures of food in magazines and on TV, and many of my recipes are created because I saw something that looked delicious, then figured out how to make a quick, healthy version that tasted as good as it looked!

When I have time for "recreational reading," I also love to look through church and community cookbooks. I read recipes as if I were reading a novel. When something grabs my attention, I ask, "How can I have this taste the way it's supposed to but get rid of most of the fats, sugars, and sodium (and make it easier in the process)?"

Sometimes just the name of a recipe intrigues me enough to come up with something new. I dream about how a recipe with that name ought to taste, and then I envision the ingredients and preparation to do the trick.

Dining Well Even without a Recipe

Do I cook up every meal—even breakfast—from one of my recipes? *Of course not!* Sometimes I am so rushed, I have cereal and milk for breakfast. But it's never just plain cereal and just plain skim milk. One morning I might have corn flakes with a tiny finger banana sliced over the cereal, then sprinkle two teaspoons of chopped pecans and a tablespoon of raisins on top. When I add skim milk and sugar substitute, I've got a feast-in-a-bowl to crunch on.

Freezer waffles can be a great choice. In fact, anything that's quick, easy, and healthy is worth giving a try. One thing I do often when I make pancakes is double the recipe, make extra pancakes and freeze them, then microwave them on a busy morning. Bisquick Reduced-Fat mix or Aunt Jemima Lite Pancake Mix are both great choices. The thing that takes the most time in making pancakes is getting the griddle hot enough the first time. Once you do, you might as well make a few extra pancakes and save them for when you're on the run. The texture is good, and they come out of the microwave tasting almost as if they'd just come off the griddle.

Trading Sugar and Fat for Flavor with Spice

Currently, many "healthy" recipes concentrate on eliminating the fats—and ignore the excess sugars in food. My recipes will *always* be both low fat and low sugar. Many people must watch sugar intake as much as fat because of diabetes, hypoglycemia, or triglyceride concerns, and for those who want to lose weight, watching both fat and sugar is a *must.*

One of the ways I increase flavor in my healthy recipes is with spices. I tend to stay in the middle of the road when it comes to the amount of spice I use. Those of you who prefer to live on the spicier side of life will probably want to add to the amount of spice I use, even double it in some recipes. And those who prefer a tamer flavor might want to start with about half of what I suggest the first time you try something. It's up to you to personalize these recipes according to your needs—*instead* of feeling you must prepare them exactly as I do.

Well, now you know most of my secrets for creating healthy recipes—and you're ready to begin creating your own. Don't give up when there's a flavor or dish you really want to transform into a healthy version; if you just can't solve the mystery, please send it to me for HELP!

Fourteen

The Healthy Exchanges Kitchen

If you ever come to DeWitt, Iowa, and visit the Lunds, I can already guess your reaction when you see where I've cooked up thousands of Healthy Exchanges recipes. You'll be surprised to discover I don't have a massive test kitchen stocked with every modern appliance and handy gadget ever made. My tiny galley kitchen has room for only one person at a time, but it hasn't stopped me from feeling the sky's the limit when it comes to seeking out great healthy taste!

Because storage is at such a premium in my "test kitchen," I don't waste space with equipment I don't really need. Here's a list of what I consider worth having. If you notice serious gaps in your equipment, you can probably find most of what you need at a local discount store or garage sale. If your kitchen is equipped with more sophisticated appliances, don't feel guilty about using them. Enjoy every appliance you can find room for or that you can afford. Just be assured that healthy, quick, and delicious food can be prepared with the "basics."

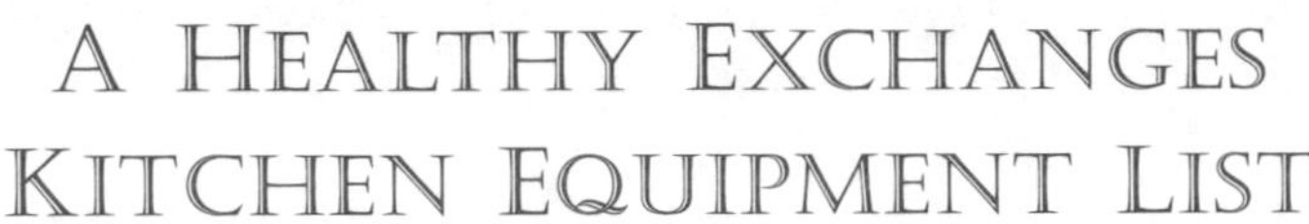

A Healthy Exchanges Kitchen Equipment List

Good-quality nonstick skillets (medium, large)
Good-quality saucepans (small, medium, large)
Glass mixing bowls (small, medium, large)
Glass measures for liquid ingredients (1 cup, 2 cup, 4 cup, 8 cup)
Sharp knives (paring, chef, butcher)
Rubber spatulas
Wire whisks
Measuring spoons
Measuring cups for dry ingredients
Large mixing spoons
Egg separator
Covered jar
Vegetable parer
Grater
Potato masher
Electric mixer
Electric blender
Electric skillet
Cooking timer
Slow cooker
Air popper for popcorn
Kitchen scales (unless you always use my recipes)
Wire racks for cooling baked goods
Electric toaster oven (to conserve energy for those times when only one item is being baked or for a recipe that requires a short baking time)
4-inch round custard dishes
Glass pie plates
8-by-8-inch glass baking dishes
Cake pans (9-by-9-, 9-by-13-inch)
10¾-by-7-by-1½-inch biscuit pan
Cookie sheets (good nonstick ones)
Jelly-roll pan
Muffin tins
5-by-9-inch bread pan
Plastic colander
Cutting board
Pie wedge server
Square-shaped server
Can opener (I prefer manual)
Rolling pin

How to Read a Healthy Exchanges® Recipe

The Healthy Exchanges Nutritional Analysis

Before using these recipes, you may wish to consult your physician or health-care provider to be sure they are appropriate for you. The information in this book is not intended to take the place of any medical advice. It reflects my experiences, studies, research, and opinions regarding healthy eating.

Each recipe includes nutritional information calculated in three ways:

Healthy Exchanges Weight Loss Choices™ or Exchanges (HE)
Calories, fiber and fat grams
Diabetic exchanges

In every Healthy Exchanges recipe, the Diabetic Exchanges have been calculated by a registered dietitian. All the other calculations were done by computer, using the Food Processor II software. When the ingredient listing gives more than one choice, the first ingredient listed is the one used in the recipe analysis. Due to inevitable variations in the ingredients you choose to use, the nutritional values should be considered approximate.

The annotation "(limited)" following Protein counts in some recipes indicates that consumption of whole eggs should be limited to four per week.

Please note the following symbols:

☆ This star means read the recipe's direction carefully for special instructions about division of ingredients.

❄ This symbol indicates FREEZES WELL.

South St. Paul Public Library
106 Third Avenue North
South St. Paul, MN 55075

Fifteen

A Few Rules for Success

A very important part of any journey is knowing where you are going and the best way to get there. If you plan and prepare before you start to cook, you should reach mealtime with foods to write home about!

1. **Read the entire recipe from start to finish** and be sure you understand the process involved. Check that you have all the equipment you will need *before* you begin.
2. **Check the ingredient list** and be sure you have *everything* and in the amounts required. (Keep cooking sprays handy—while they're not listed as ingredients, I use them all the time.)
3. **Set out *all* the ingredients and equipment needed** to prepare the recipe on the counter near you *before* you start. Remember that old saying, *A stitch in time saves nine.* It applies in the kitchen, too.

4. **Do as much advance preparation as possible** before actually cooking. Chop, cut, grate, or whatever is needed to prepare the ingredients and have them ready before you start to mix. Turn the oven on at least 10 minutes before putting food in to bake, to allow the oven to preheat to the proper temperature.

5. **Use a kitchen timer** to tell you when the cooking or baking time is up. Because stove temperatures vary slightly by manufacturer, you may want to set your timer for 5 minutes less than the suggested time just to prevent overcooking. Check the progress of your dish at that time, then decide if you need the additional minutes or not.

6. **Measure carefully.** Use glass measures for liquids and metal or plastic cups for dry ingredients. My recipes are based on standard measurements. Unless I tell you it's a scant or full cup, measure the cup level.

7. **For best results, follow the recipe instructions exactly.** Feel free to substitute ingredients that *don't change* the basic chemistry of the recipe, but be sure to leave key ingredients alone. For example, you could substitute sugar-free instant *chocolate* pudding for sugar-free *butterscotch* instant pudding, but if you used a 6-serving package when a 4-serving package was listed in the ingredients, or you used instant when cook-and-serve is required, you won't get the right result.

8. **Clean up as you go.** It is much easier to wash a few items at a time than to face a whole counterful of dirty dishes later. The same is true for spills on the counter or floor.

9. **Be careful about doubling or halving a recipe.** Though many recipes can be altered successfully to serve more or fewer people, *many cannot.* This is especially true when it comes to spices and liquids. If you try to double a recipe that calls for 1 teaspoon pumpkin-pie spice, for example, and you double the spice, you may end up with a too-spicy taste. I usually suggest increasing spices or liquid by 1½ times when doubling a recipe. If it tastes a little bland to you, you can increase the spice to 1¾ times the original amount the next time you prepare the dish. Remember: You can

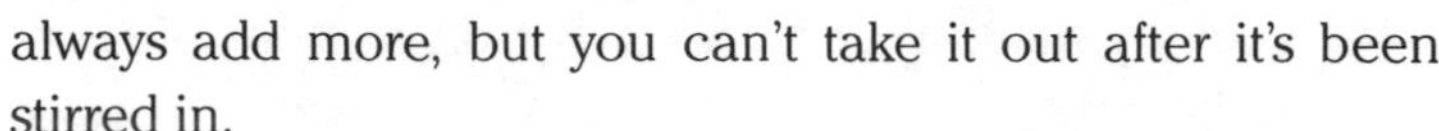

always add more, but you can't take it out after it's been stirred in.

The same is true with liquid ingredients. If you wanted to triple a recipe like my Italian Loose Meat Sandwiches because you were planning to serve a crowd, you might think you should use three times as much of every ingredient. Don't, or you could end up with Loose Meat Soup! The original recipe calls for 1 cup of tomato sauce, so I'd suggest using 2 cups of sauce when you triple the recipe (or 1½ cups if you double it). You'll still have a good-tasting sandwich that won't run all over the plate.

10. **Write your reactions next to each recipe once you've served it.**

    Yes, that's right. I'm giving you permission to write in this book. It's yours, after all. Ask yourself: Did everyone like it? Did you have to add another half teaspoon of chili seasoning to please your family, who like to live on the spicier side of the street? You may even want to rate the recipe on a scale of 1 ☆ to 4 ☆, depending on what you thought of it. (Four stars would be the top rating—and I hope you'll feel that way about many of my recipes.) Jotting down your comments while they are fresh in your mind will help you personalize the recipe to your own taste the next time you prepare it.

My Best Healthy Exchanges Tips and Tidbits

Measurements, General Cooking Tips, and Basic Ingredients

The word **moderation** best describes **my use of fats, sugar substitutes,** and **sodium** in these recipes. Wherever possible, I've used cooking spray for sautéing and for browning meats and vegetables. I also use reduced-calorie margarine and no-fat mayonnaise and salad dressings. Lean ground turkey *or* ground beef can be used in the recipes. Just be sure whatever you choose is at least *90 percent lean.*

I've also included **small amounts of sugar and brown-sugar substitutes as the sweetening agent** in many of the recipes. I don't drink a hundred cans of soda a day or eat enough artificially sweetened foods in a twenty-four-hour time period to be troubled by sugar substitutes. But if this is a concern of yours and you *do not* need to watch your sugar intake, you can always replace the sugar substitutes with processed sugar and the sugar-free products with regular ones.

I created my recipes knowing they would also be used by hypoglycemics, diabetics, and those concerned about triglycerides. If you choose to use sugar instead, be sure to count the additional calories.

A word of caution when cooking with **sugar substitutes:** Use **saccharin-based** sweeteners when **heating or baking.** In recipes that **don't require heat, aspartame** (known as Nutrasweet) works well in uncooked dishes but leaves an aftertaste in baked products.

I'm often asked why I use an **8-by-8-inch baking dish** in my recipes. It's for portion control. If the recipe says it serves 4, just cut down the center, turn the dish, and cut again. Like magic, there's your serving. Also, if this is the only recipe you are preparing that requires an oven, the square dish fits into a tabletop toaster oven easily to save energy.

To make life even easier, **whenever a recipe calls for ounce measurements** (other than raw meats) I've included the closest cup equivalent. I need to use my scale daily when creating recipes, so I've measured for you at the same time.

Most of the recipes are for **4 to 6 servings.** If you don't have that many to feed, do what I do: freeze individual portions. Then all you have to do is choose something from the freezer and take it to work for lunch or have your evening meals prepared in advance for the week. In this way, I always have something on hand that is both good to eat and good for me. (When freezing, be sure to label your individual portion for easy identification.)

Unless a recipe includes hard-boiled eggs, cream cheese, mayonnaise, or a raw vegetable, **the leftovers should freeze well.** (I've marked recipes that freeze well with the symbol of a

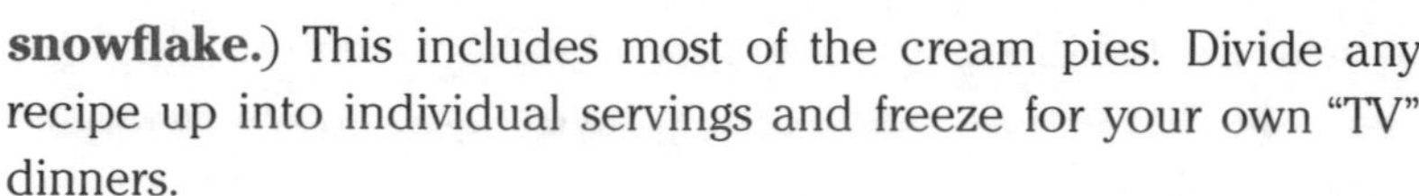

snowflake.) This includes most of the cream pies. Divide any recipe up into individual servings and freeze for your own "TV" dinners.

Unless I specify **"covered"** for simmering or baking, prepare my recipes **uncovered.** Occasionally you will read a recipe that asks you to cover a dish for a time, then to uncover it, so read the directions carefully to avoid confusion—and to get the best results.

Low-fat cooking spray is another blessing in a Healthy Exchanges kitchen. It's currently available in three flavors . . .

- **Olive-oil flavored** when cooking Mexican, Italian, or Greek dishes
- **Butter flavored** when the hint of butter is desired
- **Regular** for everything else.

A quick spray of butter-flavored spray makes air-popped popcorn a low-fat taste treat, or try it as a butter substitute on steaming hot corn on the cob. One light spray of the skillet when browning meat will convince you that you're using "old-fashioned fat," and a quick coating of the casserole dish before you add the ingredients will make serving easier and cleanup quicker.

I use **reduced-sodium canned chicken broth** in place of dry bouillon to lower the sodium content. The intended flavor is still present in the prepared dish. As a reduced-sodium beef broth is not currently available (at least not in DeWitt, Iowa), I use the canned regular beef broth. The sodium content is still lower than regular dry bouillon.

Whenever **cooked rice or pasta** is an ingredient, follow the package directions, but eliminate the salt and/or margarine called for. This helps lower the sodium and fat content. It tastes just fine; trust me on this.

Proteins

I use **eggs** in moderation. I enjoy the real thing on an average of three to four times a week. So, my recipes are calculated on using whole eggs. However, if you choose to use egg substitute, the finished product will turn out just fine and the fat grams per serving will be even lower than those listed.

If you like the look, taste, and feel of **hard-boiled eggs** in salads but haven't been using them because of the cholesterol in the yolk, I have a couple of alternatives for you: 1) Pour an 8-ounce carton of egg substitute into a medium skillet sprayed with cooking spray. Cover skillet tightly and cook over low heat until substitute is just set, about 10 minutes. Remove from heat and let set, still covered, for 10 minutes more. Uncover and cool completely. Chop set mixture. This will make about 1 cup of chopped egg. 2) Even easier is to hard-boil real eggs, toss the yolk away, and chop the white. Either way, you don't deprive yourself of the pleasure of egg in your salad.

In most recipes calling for **egg substitutes,** you can use 2 egg whites in place of the equivalent of 1 egg substitute. Just break the eggs open and toss the yolks away. I can hear some of you already saying, "But that's wasteful!" Well, take a look at the price on the egg substitute package (which usually has the equivalent of 4 eggs in it), then look at the price of a dozen eggs, from which you'd get the equivalent of 6 egg substitutes. Now, what's wasteful about that?

Whenever I include **cooked chicken** in a recipe, I use roasted white meat without skin. Whenever I include **roast beef or pork** in a recipe, I use the loin cuts because they are much leaner. However, most of the time, I do my roasting of all these meats at the local deli. I just ask for a chunk of their lean roasted meat, 6 or 8 ounces, and ask them not to slice it. When I get home, I cube or dice the meat and am ready to use it in my recipe. The reason I do this is threefold: 1) I'm getting just the amount I need without leftovers; 2) I don't have the expense of heating the oven; and 3) I'm not throwing away the bone, gristle, and fat I'd be cutting away from the meat. Overall, it is probably cheaper to "roast" it the way I do.

Did you know that you can make an acceptable meat loaf without using egg for the binding? Just replace every egg with ¼ cup of liquid. You could use beef broth, tomato sauce, even applesauce, to name just a few alternatives. For a meat loaf to serve 6, I always use 1 pound of extra-lean ground beef or turkey, 6 tablespoons of dried fine bread crumbs, and ¼ cup of the liquid, plus anything else healthy that strikes my fancy at the time. I mix well and place

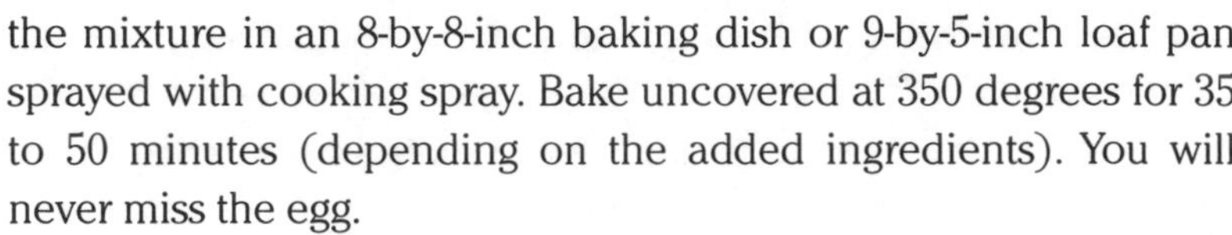

the mixture in an 8-by-8-inch baking dish or 9-by-5-inch loaf pan sprayed with cooking spray. Bake uncovered at 350 degrees for 35 to 50 minutes (depending on the added ingredients). You will never miss the egg.

Anytime you are **browning ground meat** for a casserole and want to get rid of almost all the excess fat, just place the uncooked meat loosely in a plastic colander. Set the colander in a glass pie plate. Place in microwave and cook on HIGH for 3 to 6 minutes (depending on the amount being browned), stirring often. Use as you would for any casserole. You can also chop up onions and brown them with the meat if you want.

For **gravy** with all the "old time" flavor but without the extra fat, try this almost effortless way to prepare it. (It's just about as easy as opening up a store-bought jar.) Pour the juice off your roasted meat, then set the roast aside to "rest" for about 20 minutes. Place the juice in an uncovered cake pan or other large flat pan (we want the large air surface to speed up the cooling process) and put in the freezer until the fat congeals on top and you can skim it off. Or, if you prefer, use a skimming pitcher purchased at your kitchen gadget store. Either way, measure about 1½ cups skimmed broth and pour into a medium saucepan. Cook over medium heat until heated through, about 5 minutes. In a covered jar, combine ½ cup water or cooled potato broth with 3 tablespoons flour. Shake well. Pour flour mixture into warmed juice. Combine well using a wire whisk. Continue cooking until gravy thickens, about 5 minutes. Season with salt and pepper to taste.

Why did I use flour instead of cornstarch? Because any leftovers will reheat nicely with the flour base and would not with a cornstarch base. Also, 3 tablespoons of flour works out to 1 Bread/Starch exchange. This virtually fat-free gravy makes about 2 cups, so you could spoon about ½ cup gravy on your low-fat mashed potatoes and only have to count your gravy as a ¼ Bread/Starch exchange.

Milk and Yogurt

Take it from me—nonfat dry milk powder is great! I *do not* use it for drinking, but I *do* use it for cooking. Here are three good reasons why:

1. It is very **inexpensive.**

2. It **does not sour** because you use it only as needed. Store the box in your refrigerator or freezer and it will keep almost forever.

3. You can easily **add extra calcium** to just about any recipe without added liquid.

I consider nonfat dry milk powder one of the modern-day miracles of convenience. But do purchase a good national name brand (I like Carnation), and keep it fresh by proper storage.

In many of my pies and puddings, I use nonfat dry milk powder and water instead of skim milk. Usually I call for ⅔ cup nonfat dry milk powder and 1¼ to 1½ cups water or liquid. In this way I can get the nutrients of two cups of milk but much less liquid, and the end result is much creamier. Also, the recipe sets up more quickly, usually in 5 minutes or less. So if someone knocks on your door unexpectedly at mealtime, you can quickly throw a pie together and enjoy it minutes later.

You can make your own **"sour cream"** by combining ¾ cup plain fat-free yogurt with ⅓ cup nonfat dry milk powder. The dry milk stabilizes the yogurt and keeps the whey from separating, helps to cut the tartness of the yogurt, increases the calcium by 100 percent, and is virtually fat-free. Isn't it great how we can make that distant relative of sour cream a first kissin' cousin by adding the nonfat dry milk powder? Or, if you place 1 cup of plain fat-free yogurt in a sieve lined with a coffee filter and put the sieve over a small bowl and refrigerate for about 6 hours, you will end up with a very good alternative to sour cream.

To **stabilize yogurt** when cooking or baking with it, just add 1 teaspoon of cornstarch to every ¾ cup yogurt.

If a recipe calls for **evaporated skim milk** and you don't have any in the cupboard, make your own. For every ½ cup evaporated skim milk needed, combine ⅓ cup nonfat dry milk powder and ½ cup water. Use as you would evaporated skim milk.

You can also make your own **sugar-free and fat-free sweet-**

ened condensed milk at home. Combine 1⅓ cups nonfat dry milk powder and ½ cup cold water in a 2-cup glass measure. Cover and microwave on HIGH until mixture is hot but *not* boiling. Stir in ½ cup Sprinkle Sweet or Sugar Twin. Cover and refrigerate for at least 4 hours. This mixture will keep for up to two weeks in the refrigerator. Use in just about any recipe that calls for sweetened condensed milk.

For any recipe that calls for **buttermilk,** you might want to try Jo's Buttermilk: Blend one cup of water and ⅔ cup dry milk powder (the nutrients are equal to two cups of skim milk). Add 2 teaspoons white vinegar and stir, then let it sit for at least 10 minutes.

One of my subscribers was looking for a way to further restrict salt intake and needed a substitute for **cream of mushroom soup.** For many of my recipes, I use Healthy Request Cream of Mushroom Soup, as it is a reduced-sodium product. The label suggests two servings per can, but I usually incorporate the soup into a recipe serving at least four. By doing this, I've reduced the sodium in the soup by half again.

But if you must restrict your sodium even more, try making my Healthy Exchanges **Creamy Mushroom Sauce.** Place 1½ cups evaporated skim milk and 3 tablespoons flour in a covered jar. Shake well and pour mixture into a medium saucepan sprayed with butter-flavored cooking spray. Add ½ cup canned sliced mushrooms, rinsed and drained. Cook over medium heat, stirring often, until mixture thickens. Add any seasonings of your choice. You can use this sauce in any recipe that calls for one 10¾-ounce can of cream of mushroom soup.

Why did I choose these proportions and ingredients?

- 1½ cups of evaporated skim milk is the amount in one can.
- It's equal to three Milk Choices or exchanges.
- It's the perfect amount of liquid and flour for a medium cream sauce.
- 3 tablespoons of flour is equal to one Bread/Starch choice or exchange.
- A flour-based sauce will reheat beautifully (which is not the case with a cornstarch-based sauce).
- The mushrooms are one Vegetable Choice or exchange.
- This sauce is virtually fat free, sugar free, and sodium free.

Fruits and Vegetables

If you want to enjoy a **"fruit shake"** with some pizazz, just combine soda water and unsweetened fruit juice in a blender. Add crushed ice. Blend on HIGH until thick. Refreshment without guilt.

You'll see that many recipes use ordinary **canned vegetables.** They're much cheaper than reduced-sodium versions, and once you rinse and drain them, the sodium is reduced anyway. I believe in saving money wherever possible so we can afford the best fat-free and sugar-free products as they come onto the market.

All three kinds of **vegetables—fresh, frozen, and canned**—have their place in a healthy diet. My husband, Cliff, hates the taste of frozen or fresh green beans, thinks the texture is all wrong, so I use canned green beans instead. In this case, canned vegetables have their proper place when I'm feeding my husband. If someone in your family has a similar concern, it's important to respond to it so everyone can be happy and enjoy the meal.

When I use **fruits or vegetables** like apples, cucumbers, and zucchini, I wash them really well and **leave the skin on.** It provides added color, fiber, and attractiveness to any dish. And, because I use processed flour in my cooking, I like to increase the fiber in my diet by eating my fruits and vegetables in their closest-to-natural state.

The next time you warm up canned vegetables such as carrots or green beans, drain the liquid from the can and heat the vegetables in ¼ cup beef or chicken broth. It gives a nice variation to an old standby.

Here's a simple **white sauce** for vegetables and casseroles that can be made without adding fat by spraying a medium saucepan with butter-flavored cooking spray. Place 1½ cups evaporated skim milk and 3 tablespoons flour into a covered jar. Shake well. Pour into sprayed saucepan and cook over medium heat until thick, stirring constantly. Add salt and pepper to taste. You can also add ½ cup canned drained mushrooms and/or 3 ounces (¾ cup) shredded reduced-fat cheese. Continue cooking until cheese melts.

Zip up canned or frozen green beans with **chunky salsa:** ½ cup to 2 cups beans. Heat thoroughly. Chunky salsa also makes a wonderful dressing on lettuce salads. It only counts as a vegetable, so enjoy.

Thaw light whipped topping in the refrigerator overnight. Never try to force the thawing by stirring or using a microwave to soften. Stirring it will remove the air from the topping that gives it the lightness and texture we want, and there's not enough fat in it to survive being heated.

Many of my dessert recipes call for a frosting of whipped topping, but use *only* one half cup! For best results, use a good brand. I use Cool Whip Lite or La Creme Lite. Make sure the topping is fully thawed. Always spread from the center to the sides using a rubber spatula. This way, ½ cup topping will literally cover an entire pie. Remember, the operative word is *frost,* not pile the entire container on top of the pie!

Here's a way to extend the flavor (and oils) of purchased whipped topping. Blend together ¾ cup plain nonfat yogurt and ⅓ cup nonfat dry milk powder. Add sugar substitute to equal 2 tablespoons sugar, 1 cup Cool Whip Lite, and 1 teaspoon of the flavoring of your choice (vanilla, coconut, or almond are all good choices). *Gently* mix by hand and use as you would whipped topping. The texture is almost a cross between marshmallow cream and whipped cream. This is enough to mound high on a pie.

For a different taste when preparing sugar-free instant pudding mixes, use ¾ cup plain fat-free yogurt for one of the required cups of milk. Blend as usual. It will be *thicker and creamier.* And, no, it doesn't taste like yogurt. Another variation for the sugar-free instant vanilla pudding is to use 1 cup skim milk and 1 cup crushed pineapple with juice. Mix as usual.

For a special treat that tastes anything but "diet," try placing **spreadable fruit** in a container and microwave for about 15 seconds. Then pour the melted fruit spread over a serving of nonfat ice cream or frozen yogurt. One tablespoon of spreadable fruit is equal to 1 fruit serving. Some combinations to get you started are apricot over chocolate ice cream, strawberry over strawberry ice cream, or any flavor over vanilla. Another way I use spreadable fruit is to make a delicious **topping for a cheesecake or angel food cake.** I blend ½ cup of fruit and ½ cup Cool Whip Lite with a teaspoon of coconut extract.

The next time you are making treats for the family, try using **unsweetened applesauce** for some or all of the required oil in the recipe. For instance, if the recipe calls for ½ cup cooking oil, use *up to the ½ cup* in applesauce. It works and most people will not even notice the difference. It's great in purchased cake mixes, but so far I haven't been able to figure out a way to deep-fat fry with it!

Many people have experimented with my tip about **substituting applesauce and artificial sweetener for butter and sugar,** but what if you aren't satisfied with the result? One woman wrote to me about a recipe for her grandmother's cookies that called for 1 cup butter and 1½ cups sugar. Well, any recipe that depends on as much butter and sugar as this one does is generally not a good candidate for "healthy exchanges." The original recipe needed a large quantity of fat to produce the crisp cookie just like the one Grandma made.

Unsweetened applesauce can be used to substitute for vegetable oil with various degrees of success, but not to replace butter, lard, or margarine. If your recipe calls for ½ cup oil or less, and it's a quick bread, muffin, or bar cookie, it should work to replace the oil with applesauce. If the recipe calls for more than ½ cup oil, then experiment with half oil, half applesauce. You've still made the recipe healthier, even if you haven't removed all the oil from it.

Another rule for healthy substitution: Up to ½ cup sugar or less can be replaced by *an artificial sweetener that can withstand the heat of baking,* like Sprinkle Sweet or Sugar Twin. If it requires more than ½ cup sugar, cut the amount needed by 75 percent and use ½ cup sugar substitute and sugar for the rest. Other options: Reduce the butter and sugar by 25 percent and see if the finished product still satisfies you in taste and appearance. Or, make the cookies just as Grandma did, realizing they are part of your family's holiday tradition. Enjoy a moderate serving of a couple of cookies once or twice during the season, and just forget about them the rest of the year.

Another trick I often use is to include tiny amounts of "real-people" food, such as coconut, but extend the flavor by using extracts. Try it—you will be surprised by how little of the real thing you can use and still feel you are not being deprived.

If you are preparing a pie filling that has ample moisture, just line the bottom of a 9-by-9-inch cake pan with dry **graham crackers.** Pour the filling over the top of the crackers. Cover and refrigerate until the moisture has enough time to soften the crackers.

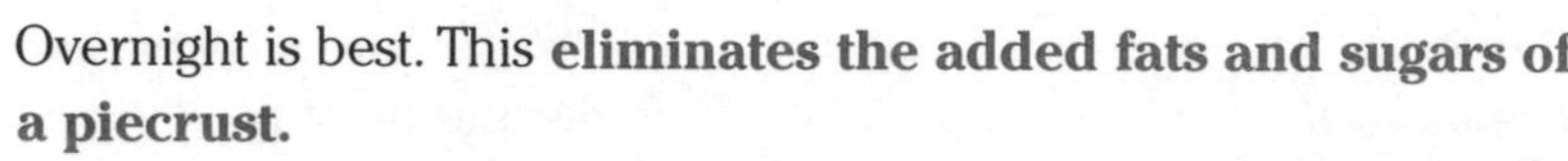

Overnight is best. This **eliminates the added fats and sugars of a piecrust.**

Many of my pie recipes can be frozen (always check for the ❄ symbol to be sure) but it's best to cut the leftover pie into individual servings and insert them in individual freezer bags before you place them in the freezer. That way, when you need one piece, you don't have to thaw the entire pie. If you freeze and thaw a pie more than once, you could end up with a substandard result—and a disappointing dessert!

When **stirring fat-free cream cheese to soften it,** use only a sturdy spoon, *never an electric mixer.* The speed of a mixer can cause the cream cheese to lose its texture and become watery.

Did you know you can make your own **fruit-flavored yogurt**? Mix 1 tablespoon of any flavor of spreadable fruit spread with ¾ cup plain yogurt. It's every bit as tasty and much cheaper. You can also make your own **lemon yogurt** by combining 3 cups plain fat-free yogurt with 1 tub Crystal Light lemonade powder. Mix well, cover, and store in refrigerator. I think you will be pleasantly surprised by the ease, cost, and flavor of this "made from scratch" calcium-rich treat. P.S.: You can make any flavor you like by using any of the Crystal Light mixes—Cranberry? Iced tea? You decide.

Sugar-free puddings and gelatins are important to many of my recipes, but if you prefer to avoid sugar substitutes, you can prepare the recipes with regular puddings or gelatins. The calories will be higher, but you will still be cooking low-fat.

When a recipe calls for **chopped nuts** (and you only have whole ones), who wants to dirty the food processor just for a couple of tablespoonsful? You could try to chop them using your cutting board, but be prepared for bits and pieces to fly all over the kitchen. I use "Grandma's food processor": In a small glass bowl, I chop the biggest nuts I can find using a metal biscuit cutter.

If you have a **leftover muffin** and are looking for something a little different for breakfast, you can make a **"breakfast sundae."** Crumble the muffin into a cereal bowl. Sprinkle a serving of fresh fruit over it and top with a couple of tablespoons of nonfat plain yogurt sweetened with sugar substitute and your choice of extract. The thought of it just might make you jump out of bed with a smile on your face. (Speaking of muffins, did you know that if you fill the unused muffin wells with water when baking muffins, you help ensure more even baking and protect the muffin pan at the same time?)

The secret of making **good meringues** without sugar is to use 1 tablespoon of Sprinkle Sweet or Sugar Twin for every egg white, and a small amount of extract. Use ½ to 1 teaspoon for the batch. Almond, vanilla, and coconut are all good choices. Use the same amount of cream of tartar you usually do. Bake the meringue in the same old way. Don't think you can't have meringue pies because you can't eat sugar. You can, if you do it my way. (Remember that egg whites whip up best at room temperature.)

Homemade or Store-bought?

I've been asked which is better for you, homemade from scratch, or purchased foods. My answer is *both!* They each have a place in a healthy lifestyle.

Take **piecrusts,** for instance. If you love spending your spare time in the kitchen preparing foods, and you're using low-fat, low-sugar, and reasonably low-sodium ingredients, go for it! But if, like so many people, your time is limited and you've learned to read labels, you could be better off using purchased foods.

I know that when I prepare a pie (and I experiment with a couple of pies each week, because this is Cliff's favorite dessert), I use a purchased crust. Why? Mainly because I can't make a good-tasting piecrust that is lower in fat than the brands I use. Also, purchased piecrusts fit my rule of "If it takes longer to fix than to eat, forget it!"

I've checked the nutrient information for the purchased piecrust against recipes for traditional and "diet" piecrusts, using my computer software program. The purchased crust calculated lower in both fat and calories! I have tried some low-fat and low-sugar recipes, but they just didn't spark my taste buds or were so complicated you needed an engineering degree just to get the crust in the pie plate.

I'm very happy with the purchased piecrusts in my recipes, because the finished product rarely, if ever, has more than 30 percent of total calories coming from fat. I also believe that we have to prepare foods our families and friends will eat with us on a regular basis and not feel deprived, or we've wasted time, energy, and money.

I could use a purchased "lite" **pie filling,** but instead I make my own. Here I can save both fat and sugar and still make the filling

almost as fast as opening a can. The bottom line: Know what you have to "spend" when it comes to both time and fat/sugar calories, then make the best decision you can for you and your family. And don't go without an occasional piece of pie because you think it isn't *necessary.* A delicious pie prepared in a healthy way is one of the simple pleasures of life. It's a little thing, but it can make all the difference between just getting by with the bare minimum and leading a full and healthy lifestyle.

I'm sure you'll add to this list of cooking tips as you begin preparing Healthy Exchanges recipes and discover how easy it can be to adapt your own favorite recipes using these ideas and your own common sense.

Making Healthy Exchanges Eating Work for You

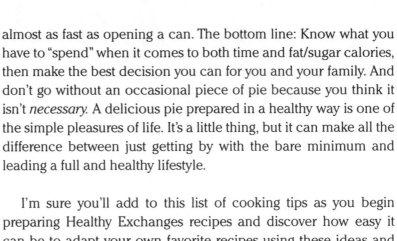

You're ready now to begin a wonderful journey to better health. In the preceding pages, you've discovered the remarkable variety of good food available to you when you begin eating the Healthy Exchanges way. You've stocked your pantry and learned many of my food preparation "secrets" that will point you on the way to delicious success.

But before you head for the recipes, I'd like to share a few tips that I've learned while traveling that have led to healthier eating habits. It took me a long time to learn how to eat *smarter.* In fact, I'm still working on it. But I am getting better. For years, I could *inhale* a five-course meal in five minutes flat—and still make room for a second helping of dessert!

Now I follow certain signposts on the road that guide me on the right path. I hope these ideas will help point you in the right direction as well.

1. **Eat slowly** so your brain has time to catch up with your tummy. Cut and chew each bite deliberately. Try putting your fork down between bites. Stop eating as soon as you

feel full. Crumple up your napkin and throw it on top of your plate so you don't continue to eat when you are no longer hungry.

2. **Smaller plates** may help you feel more satisfied by your food portions *and* limit the amount you can put on the plate.
3. **Watch portion size.** If you are *truly* hungry, you can always add more food to your plate once you've finished your initial serving. But remember to count the additional food accordingly.
4. **Always eat at your dining room or kitchen table.** You deserve better than nibbling from an open refrigerator or over the sink. Make an attractive place setting, even if you're eating alone. Feed your eyes as well as your stomach. By always eating at a table, you will become much more aware of your true food intake. For some reason, many of us conveniently "forget" the food we swallow while standing over the stove, munching in the car, or on the run.
5. **Avoid doing anything else while you are eating.** If you read the paper or watch television while you eat, it's easy to consume too much food without realizing it, because you are concentrating on something else besides what you're eating. Then, when you look down at your plate and see that it's empty, you wonder where all the food went and why you still feel hungry.

Day by day, as you travel the road to good health, it will become easier to make the right choices, to eat *smarter.* But don't ever deceive yourself into thinking that you'll be able to put your eating habits on cruise control and forget about them. Making a commitment to eat good healthy food and sticking to it takes some effort. But with all the good-tasting recipes in this book, just think how well you're going to eat—and enjoy it—from now on!

Healthy, Lean Bon Appetit!

Jo Anna

The Recipes

Soups

Chinese Egg Drop Soup

French Onion Soup

Iowa Corn Chowder

Italian Tomato Rice Soup

Italian Zucchini Tomato Soup

Lifesaver Soup

Onion Noodle Soup

Quick Chicken Soup

Southwestern Vegetable Soup

Tex-Mex Calico Corn Chili

Chinese Egg Drop Soup

Serves 2 (1 cup)

My son James *loves* Egg Drop Soup and will not settle for anything but the best. He gives my version two soup spoons up, and it cooks up faster than you can drive to the nearest Chinese restaurant!

2 cups (one 16-ounce can) Campbell's Healthy Request chicken broth
1 teaspoon chopped dried chives
½ cup frozen peas
1 teaspoon reduced-calorie margarine
1 egg, beaten, or *equivalent in egg substitute*

In a medium saucepan, heat broth until hot but not boiling. Add chives, peas, and margarine. Cook 2 to 3 minutes. Stir in beaten egg. Continue cooking until egg starts to set. Serve at once.

Each serving equals:

HE: ½ Protein (limited) • ½ Bread • ¼ Fat • 16 Optional Calories

83 Calories • 3 gm Fat • 8 gm Protein • 6 gm Carbohydrate • 441 mg Sodium • 0 gm Fiber

DIABETIC: ½ Meat • ½ Starch

French Onion Soup

Serves 2 (1 full cup)

This hearty soup can trace its heritage back to peasant stock but tastes as good as any found in the fanciest French restaurant. It's up to you whether you let anyone know just how easy it is to prepare.

1½ cups thinly sliced onion
1¾ cups (one 15-ounce can) canned beef broth
½ teaspoon Worcestershire sauce
3 slices reduced-calorie white bread, toasted and cubed
2 tablespoons grated Kraft House Italian or *Parmesan cheese*

In a medium saucepan sprayed with butter-flavored cooking spray, lightly brown onion. Add beef broth and Worcestershire sauce. Cover and simmer 10 minutes or until onion is tender. Remove from heat. In a covered bowl, mix together cubed toast and cheese. Add to onion mixture. Stir gently to combine. Serve at once.

Each serving equals:

HE: 1½ Vegetable • ¾ Bread • ¼ Protein • 18 Optional Calories

163 Calories • 3 gm Fat • 11 gm Protein • 23 gm Carbohydrate • 893 mg Sodium • 3 gm Fiber

DIABETIC: 1 Vegetable • 1 Starch • ½ Meat

Iowa Corn Chowder

Serves 4 (1⅓ cups)

This hearty soup makes a delightful change of pace for lunchtime. It keeps well in a thermos or warms up with ease in a microwave.

½ cup chopped onion
2 cups skim milk
1½ cups frozen whole-kernel corn
1 (10¾-ounce) can Campbell's Healthy Request Cream of Mushroom Soup
½ cup (one 2.5-ounce jar) canned sliced mushrooms, drained
1 cup (4 ounces) diced cooked potatoes
1 teaspoon dried parsley flakes
¼ teaspoon black pepper
2 tablespoons Hormel Bacon Bits

In a medium saucepan sprayed with butter-flavored cooking spray, sauté onion until tender, about 5 minutes. Add skim milk, corn, mushroom soup, mushrooms, potatoes, parsley flakes, and black pepper. Mix well. Continue cooking 3 minutes. Reduce heat. Stir in bacon bits. Simmer 2 to 3 minutes.

Each serving equals:

HE: 1 Bread • ½ Skim Milk • ½ Vegetable • ½ Slider • 14 Optional Calories

194 Calories • 2 gm Fat • 9 gm Protein • 35 gm Carbohydrate • 535 mg Sodium • 3 gm Fiber

DIABETIC: 2 Starch • ½ Skim Milk

Italian Tomato Rice Soup

Serves 4 (1½ cups)

This is a quick, tasty, filling, healthy, and attractive soup that blends a terrific assortment of flavors into something really special. What more can we ask for?

½ cup finely chopped onion
½ cup finely chopped green bell pepper
4 cups (two 16-ounce cans) canned tomatoes with juice
1 cup water
2 teaspoons Italian seasoning
⅛ teaspoon black pepper
¼ cup (1 ounce) chopped ripe olives
⅓ cup plus 1 tablespoon (2 ounces) chopped Canadian bacon
⅔ cup (2 ounces) dry instant rice

In a large saucepan sprayed with olive-flavored cooking spray, sauté onion and green pepper until tender. Place tomatoes and juice in blender. Blend on HIGH until pureed. Add tomatoes and water to onion and green peppers. Add Italian seasoning, black pepper, olives, and Canadian bacon. Bring mixture to a boil. Add rice; remove from heat, cover, and let set about 5 minutes.

Each serving equals:

HE: 2½ Vegetable • ½ Protein • ½ Bread • ¼ Fat

171 Calories • 3 gm Fat • 7 gm Protein • 29 gm Carbohydrate • 274 mg Sodium • 2 gm Fiber

DIABETIC: 2 Vegetable • 1 Starch • ½ Meat

Note: This is a bonus recipe, not included in any of the week's menus. Think of it as my own version of a baker's dozen—I like to give more than is expected. Besides, you can never have too many soups to choose from!

Italian Zucchini Tomato Soup

Serves 4 (full 1½ cups)

You won't recognize good old tomato soup after stirring in some zucchini and rice. This truly is a mouth-pleasing sensation, one I think you'll prepare often.

½ cup chopped onion
1 cup finely chopped zucchini
1½ cups water
1 (10¾-ounce) can Campbell's Healthy Request Tomato Soup
1¾ cups (one 15-ounce can) Hunt's Chunky Tomato Sauce
1 teaspoon Italian seasoning
⅓ cup (1 ounce) uncooked instant rice
¼ cup (¾ ounce) grated Kraft House Italian or *Parmesan cheese*

In a medium saucepan sprayed with butter-flavored cooking spray, sauté onion and zucchini for 5 minutes, stirring often. Add water, tomato soup, tomato sauce, and Italian seasoning. Mix well to combine. Bring mixture to a boil. Stir in dry rice, mixing well. Remove from heat. Cover. Let set 5 minutes; then stir gently. For each serving, spoon 1½ cups soup into a bowl and sprinkle 1 tablespoon cheese over top.

Each serving equals:
HE: 2½ Vegetable • ¼ Bread • ¼ Protein • ½ Slider • 5 Optional Calories

---

122 Calories • 2 gm Fat • 4 gm Protein • 22 gm Carbohydrate • 457 mg Sodium • 2 gm Fiber

---

DIABETIC: 2 Vegetable • 1 Starch *or* 3 Vegetable • ½ Starch

Lifesaver Soup

Serves 4 (1½ cups) ❄

A bowl of this filling soup may "save" you from reaching for unhealthy snacks. I know it has done that for me on more than one occasion. Who says you can't have soup for a quick snack break?

1½ cups Healthy Request Tomato Juice
1¾ cups (one 15-ounce can) canned beef broth
1 teaspoon Worcestershire sauce
1 cup (one 4-ounce can) canned sliced mushrooms, drained
3 cups chopped cabbage
1 cup chopped celery
¼ teaspoon lemon pepper

In a large saucepan, combine tomato juice, beef broth, Worcestershire sauce, and mushrooms. Add cabbage, celery, and lemon pepper. Cover and cook over medium heat until cabbage is tender, about 10 minutes.

Each serving equals:
HE: 3¼ Vegetable • 9 Optional Calories

---

61 Calories • 1 gm Fat • 3 gm Protein • 10 gm Carbohydrate • 486 mg Sodium • 2 gm Fiber

---

DIABETIC: 2 Vegetable

HINT: Add any veggies of *your* choice.

Onion Noodle Soup

Serves 4 (1¼ cups) ❄

I love onions and I love noodles—and I love this tasty soup. This recipe is guaranteed to put a smile on the face of any onion lover—especially because the serving size is so substantial and satisfying!

1¾ cups (one 15-ounce can) canned beef broth
2¾ cups water
1 teaspoon Worcestershire sauce
2 cups sliced onion
¾ cup mounded (1½ ounces) uncooked noodles
¼ cup (¾ ounce) grated Kraft House Italian or Parmesan cheese

In a large saucepan, combine beef broth, water, and Worcestershire sauce. Add onion. Bring mixture to a boil. Lower heat. Cover. Simmer 15 minutes. Add noodles and continue cooking until onion and noodles are tender, about 10 minutes. When serving, sprinkle 1 tablespoon cheese on top of each bowl.

Each serving equals:

HE: 1 Vegetable • ½ Bread • ¼ Protein • 18 Optional Calories

114 Calories • 2 gm Fat • 6 gm Protein • 18 gm Carbohydrate • 413 mg Sodium • 3 gm Fiber

DIABETIC: 1 Starch • ½ Vegetable • ½ Meat

Quick Chicken Soup

Serves 4 (scant 1 cup)

This is a perfect example of an "almost instant" soup that tastes like real homemade! It takes a few minutes more than just opening a store-bought can, but the payoff is downright delicious!

2 cups (one 16-ounce can) Campbell's Healthy Request Chicken Broth
1 cup water
½ cup cooked rice
¼ cup chopped sweet red pepper
2 sliced green onions
2 tablespoons chopped parsley

In a medium saucepan, combine chicken broth and water. Cover and bring mixture to boiling. Stir in cooked rice, red pepper, green onions, and parsley. Cover mixture and simmer for 3 minutes. Serve immediately.

Each serving equals:

HE: ¼ Bread • ¼ Vegetable • 8 Optional Calories

36 Calories • 0 gm Fat • 2 gm Protein • 7 gm Carbohydrate • 237 mg Sodium • 0 gm Fiber

DIABETIC: ½ Starch

HINT: ⅓ cup uncooked rice usually cooks to about ½ cup.

Southwestern Vegetable Soup

Serves 4 (1½ cups) ❄

There's a hint of Old Mexico in this updated soup. It pleases my "spice-loving guy," Cliff. I'm betting it pleases you as well. (If your taste buds demand a spicier version, add a little red pepper!)

2 cups (one 16-ounce can) canned tomatoes with juice
2 cups (one 16-ounce can) Campbell's Healthy Request Chicken Broth
1 cup shredded cabbage
½ cup chopped onion
1 cup frozen green beans
1 cup frozen carrots
2 teaspoons chili seasoning mix

Place tomatoes with juice in blender; blend on PUREE for 10 seconds. In a large saucepan, combine tomatoes, chicken broth, shredded cabbage, onion, beans, and carrots. Add chili seasoning. Bring mixture to a boil. Lower heat and simmer for 45 to 60 minutes.

Each serving equals:

HE: 2¾ Vegetable • 8 Optional Calories

77 Calories • 1 gm Fat • 4 gm Protein • 13 gm Carbohydrate • 265 mg Sodium • 1 gm Fiber

DIABETIC: 3 Vegetable or 1 Starch

Tex-Mex Calico Corn Chili

Serves 4 (1 cup) ❄

This easy chili is as satisfying as its "beefed up" cousins. More than likely, the bowls will be licked clean before anyone realizes it's meatless!

1 (10¾-ounce can Campbell's Healthy Request Tomato Soup
1 cup water
½ cup chunky salsa
10 ounces (one 16-ounce can) red kidney beans, rinsed and drained
2 cups frozen whole kernel corn
1 teaspoon chili seasoning mix
1 teaspoon dried parsley flakes

In a medium saucepan, combine tomato soup, water, and salsa. Stir in kidney beans, corn, chili seasoning mix, and parsley flakes. Cook over medium heat, stirring often, until mixture comes to a boil. Lower heat. Simmer 10 minutes.

Each serving equals:

HE: 1¼ Protein • 1 Bread • ¼ Vegetable • ¾ Slider • 2 Optional Calories

230 Calories • 2 gm Fat • 10 gm Protein • 43 gm Carbohydrate • 430 mg Sodium • 12 gm Fiber

DIABETIC: 2½ Starch • 1 Meat

Note: This is a bonus recipe, not included in any of the week's menus. Living a healthy lifestyle is full of unexpected pleasures, including extra soup recipes.

Salads

Blue Cheese Mushroom Salad

Cauliflower-Broccoli-Raisin Salad

Cottage Cheese-Stuffed Tomatoes

Deli Coleslaw

Fiesta Corn Salad

French Carrot Salad

Frisco Salad

Frosted Orange Salad

Green Bean Salad

Molded Relish Salad

Old-Style Slaw

Polynesian Carrot Salad

Quick Spinach Salad

Ranchero Vegetable Salad

Salsa Zucchini Salad

Shrimp Caesar Salad

Spinach Salad

Taffy Apple Salad

Tomato, Celery, and Cabbage Salad

Vegetable Hodgepodge Salad

Blue Cheese Mushroom Salad

Serves 4 (¾ cup)

How can we whip up a delicious yet fat-free blue cheese salad? By using fat-free dressing to impart the tangy flavor of blue cheese, that's how!

2 cups sliced fresh mushrooms
¾ cup shredded carrots
¼ cup sliced green onion
¼ cup Kraft fat-free Blue Cheese dressing
2 tablespoons Kraft fat-free mayonnaise

In a large bowl, combine mushrooms, carrots, and green onion. In a small bowl, combine blue cheese dressing and mayonnaise. Add mixture to mushroom mixture. Toss gently to combine. Cover and refrigerate at least 30 minutes. Gently stir again just before serving.

Each serving equals:

HE: 1½ Vegetable • ¼ Slider • 1 Optional Calorie

40 Calories • 0 gm Fat • 1 gm Protein • 9 gm Carbohydrate • 179 mg Sodium • 1 gm Fiber

DIABETIC: 2 Vegetable

Cauliflower-Broccoli-Raisin Salad

Serves 8 (½ cup)

This wonderful salad scored a home run with my son Tommy and me. Of course, it struck out with Cliff. If I left out the broccoli, he might give it a shot.

2¼ cups fresh cauliflower florets
2¼ cups fresh broccoli florets
½ cup chopped onion
½ cup raisins
2 tablespoons Hormel Bacon Bits
½ cup Kraft fat-free mayonnaise
2 tablespoons white vinegar
Sugar substitute to equal 2 tablespoons sugar

In a medium bowl, combine cauliflower, broccoli, onion, raisins, and bacon bits. In a small bowl, combine mayonnaise, vinegar, and sugar substitute. Pour mayonnaise mixture over vegetable mixture. Mix well to combine. Cover and refrigerate at least 2 hours. Gently stir again just before serving.

Each serving equals:

HE: 1¼ Vegetable • ½ Fruit • 18 Optional Calories

81 Calories • 1 gm Fat • 3 gm Protein • 15 gm Carbohydrate • 163 mg Sodium • 1 gm Fiber

DIABETIC: 1½ Vegetable • ½ Fruit

Cottage Cheese-Stuffed Tomatoes

Serves 2

Isn't it great when the tomato can work as the salad "bowl"? Best of all, we get to eat the "bowl" right along with the salad.

2 ripe medium tomatoes
1 cup fat-free cottage cheese
2 tablespoons chopped green bell pepper
2 tablespoons chopped green onion
½ teaspoon minced garlic
¼ teaspoon black pepper

Cut tops off tomatoes. Scoop out seeds and pulp. Turn tomatoes upside down and allow to drain 2 to 3 minutes. In a medium bowl, combine cottage cheese, green pepper, onion, garlic, and black pepper. Split tomatoes into 4 wedges, but *DO NOT* cut all the way to bottom. Evenly stuff tomatoes with cottage cheese mixture. Refrigerate at least 30 minutes.

Each serving equals:

HE: 1¼ Vegetable • 1 Protein

---

68 Calories • 0 gm Fat • 9 gm Protein • 8 gm Carbohydrate • 203 mg Sodium • 1 gm Fiber

---

DIABETIC: 1 Meat • 1 Vegetable

Deli Coleslaw

Serves 6 (⅔ cup)

If you love the type of slaw you can find in just about any delicatessen in America, then this is the slaw for you. The bits of color from the bell peppers add an appealing touch.

2½ cups shredded cabbage
¾ cup shredded carrots
¼ cup diced green bell pepper
¼ cup diced red bell pepper
¼ cup diced onion
½ cup Kraft fat-free mayonnaise
1 tablespoon white vinegar
Sugar substitute to equal 1 tablespoon sugar
2 teaspoons dried parsley flakes
¼ teaspoon black pepper

In a medium bowl, combine cabbage, carrots, green pepper, red pepper, and onion. In a small bowl, combine mayonnaise, vinegar, sugar substitute, parsley flakes, and black pepper. Add mayonnaise mixture to cabbage mixture. Mix well to combine. Cover and refrigerate at least 30 minutes. Gently stir again just before serving.

Each serving equals:

HE: 2 Vegetable • ¼ Slider • 2 Optional Calories

---

48 Calories • 0 gm Fat • 1 gm Protein • 11 gm Carbohydrate • 191 mg Sodium • 2 gm Fiber

---

DIABETIC: 1 Vegetable • 1 Free Vegetable

Fiesta Corn Salad

Serves 6 (½ cup)

Olé for the flavors of this colorful salad! I wouldn't be surprised to find you dancing around the kitchen with your sombrero on after a few bites.

2 cups frozen whole-kernel corn, thawed
¼ cup chopped red radishes
¼ cup chopped green or *white onion*
½ cup chopped green bell pepper
½ cup chunky salsa
¼ cup Kraft fat-free Ranch dressing
1 tablespoon fresh parsley
¼ teaspoon black pepper

In a medium bowl, combine corn, radishes, onion, and green pepper. Add salsa, Ranch dressing, parsley, and black pepper. Mix well to combine. Cover and refrigerate at least 30 minutes. Gently stir again just before serving.

Each serving equals:

HE: ⅔ Bread • ½ Vegetable • 13 Optional Calories

73 Calories • 1 gm Fat • 2 gm Protein • 14 gm Carbohydrate • 167 mg Sodium • 1 gm Fiber

DIABETIC: 1 Starch • ½ Vegetable

French Carrot Salad

Serves 4 (full ½ cup)

It just doesn't get any easier than this savory salad. Why not enjoy a full day's dose of beta-carotene in a bowl?

2 cups shredded carrots
½ cup diced onion
¼ cup Kraft fat-free French dressing
1 teaspoon dried parsley flakes
2 tablespoons Kraft fat-free mayonnaise

In a medium bowl, combine carrots and onion. Add French dressing, parsley, and mayonnaise. Mix gently to combine. Cover and refrigerate at least 30 minutes.

Each serving equals:

HE: 1¼ Vegetable • ¼ Slider • 3 Optional Calories

56 Calories • 0 gm Fat • 1 gm Protein • 13 gm Carbohydrate • 177 mg Sodium • 1 gm Fiber

DIABETIC: 2 Vegetable

Frisco Salad

Serves 4 (1⅓ cups)

I originally "ate" this salad with my eyes in a restaurant in San Francisco. When I returned home, I quickly re-created it in the "Healthy Exchanges Way." Who would have thought that cold beets could add so much to a salad?

4 cups shredded lettuce
1 cup (one 8-ounce can) canned beets, drained and finely diced
1 finely chopped hard-boiled egg
¼ cup Kraft fat-free Thousand Island dressing
2 teaspoons lemon juice
1 teaspoon dried parsley flakes
¼ teaspoon black pepper

In a large bowl, combine lettuce, beets, and egg. In a small bowl, combine Thousand Island dressing, lemon juice, parsley flakes, and black pepper. Add dressing mixture to lettuce mixture. Toss gently to combine. Serve at once.

Each serving equals:

HE: 2½ Vegetable • ¼ Protein (limited) • ¼ Slider

53 Calories • 1 gm Fat • 2 gm Protein • 9 gm Carbohydrate • 208 mg Sodium • 1 gm Fiber

DIABETIC: 2 Vegetable

Frosted Orange Salad

Serves 8

I just don't know of a better gelatin salad anywhere in the world! It not only pleases the mouth and tummy with its delicious citrusy flavors, its bright color is a feast for the eyes as well.

2 (4-serving) packages Jell-O sugar-free orange gelatin
1½ cups boiling water
1 cup unsweetened orange juice
1 cup (one 8-ounce can) canned crushed pineapple, packed in fruit juice, undrained
1 cup (one 11-ounce can) canned mandarin oranges, rinsed and drained
1 (4-serving) package Jell-O sugar-free lemon gelatin
1 (4-serving) package Jell-O sugar-free instant vanilla pudding mix
⅔ cup Carnation nonfat dry milk powder
1⅓ cups water
⅔ cup Cool Whip Lite

In a medium bowl, combine both packages of dry orange gelatin and boiling water. Mix well to dissolve gelatin. Add orange juice, undrained pineapple, and mandarin oranges. Mix gently to combine. Pour mixture into an 8-by-8-inch dish. Refrigerate until set, about 4 hours. In a medium bowl, combine dry lemon gelatin, dry pudding mix, and dry milk powder. Add water. Mix well using a wire whisk. Blend in Cool Whip Lite. Spread pudding mixture evenly over set gelatin mixture. Refrigerate at least 15 minutes before serving. Cut into 8 pieces.

Each serving equals:

HE: ¾ Fruit • ¼ Skim Milk • ¼ Slider • 15 Optional Calories

105 Calories • 1 gm Fat • 4 gm Protein • 20 gm Carbohydrate • 301 mg Sodium • 1 gm Fiber

DIABETIC: 1 Fruit

Green Bean Salad

Serves 4 (⅔ cup)

Crunchy, tangy, spicy, and satisfying are just a few ways to describe this easy salad. Both its appearance and flavor are guaranteed to garner you compliments.

2 cups frozen green beans, thawed
1 cup chopped fresh tomato
¼ cup chopped onion
¼ cup chopped green bell pepper
2 tablespoons Hormel Bacon Bits
¼ cup (¾ ounce) grated Kraft House Italian or *Parmesan cheese*
2 tablespoons Kraft fat-free Catalina dressing

In a large bowl, combine green beans, chopped tomato, onion, green pepper, bacon bits, and cheese. Add Catalina dressing. Toss gently to combine. Cover and refrigerate at least 30 minutes. Gently stir again just before serving.

Each serving equals:

HE: 1¾ Vegetable • ¼ Protein • ¼ Slider • 4 Optional Calories

82 Calories • 2 gm Fat • 5 gm Protein • 11 gm Carbohydrate • 227 mg Sodium • 1 gm Fiber

DIABETIC: 2 Vegetable • ½ Meat

HINT: Canned green beans, rinsed and drained, can be used instead of frozen.

Molded Relish Salad

Serves 8

This is my mother's old standby, to which I just added a few more veggies. But I know my healthier version would still meet with her approval.

1 (4-serving) package Jell-O sugar-free lime gelatin
1 cup hot water
1 cup cold water
2 tablespoons cider vinegar
1 teaspoon prepared horseradish
⅛ teaspoon black pepper
1 cup chopped cabbage
½ cup chopped cucumber
½ cup shredded carrot
2 tablespoons chopped green bell pepper
2 tablespoons chopped radishes
Lettuce leaves

In a medium bowl, combine dry gelatin and hot water. Mix well to dissolve gelatin. Add cold water, vinegar, horseradish, and black pepper. Mix gently to combine. Add cabbage, cucumber, carrot, green pepper, and radishes. Mix well. Pour mixture into an 8-by-8-inch dish. Refrigerate until set, about 4 hours. Cut into 8 pieces. When serving, place on lettuce-lined salad plates.

Each serving equals:

HE: ⅔ Vegetable • 4 Optional Calories

12 Calories • 0 gm Fat • 1 gm Protein • 2 gm Carbohydrate • 32 mg Sodium • 1 gm Fiber

DIABETIC: 1 Free Vegetable

HINT: Good topped with 1 teaspoon Kraft fat-free mayonnaise; but don't forget to count the few additional calories.

Old-Style Slaw

Serves 6 (¾ cup)

Anytime I want Cliff to do the "honey-do" jobs around our house, I just make sure I serve him a big dish of his favorite slaw. Why don't you try it with your "honey" and see if it works for you, too?

½ cup Kraft fat-free mayonnaise
2 teaspoons dried parsley flakes
1 tablespoon white vinegar
Sugar substitute to equal 2 tablespoons sugar
1 tablespoon Old Style or regular Dijon mustard
⅛ teaspoon black pepper
4 cups prepackaged coleslaw mix

In a large bowl, combine mayonnaise, parsley flakes, vinegar, sugar substitute, Old Style Dijon mustard, and black pepper. Add coleslaw mix. Mix gently to combine. Cover and refrigerate at least 1 hour. Gently stir again just before serving.

Each serving equals:

HE: 1⅓ Vegetable • 15 Optional Calories

32 Calories • 0 gm Fat • 1 gm Protein • 7 gm Carbohydrate • 164 mg Sodium • 1 gm Fiber

DIABETIC: 1 Vegetable • 1 Free Vegetable

HINT: 3½ cups shredded cabbage and ½ cup shredded carrots can be used in place of prepackaged coleslaw mix.

Polynesian Carrot Salad

Serves 4 (½ cup)

Your taste buds will think you went on vacation even if you never leave home! This flavorful salad provides a delicious blend that will remind you of warm breezes and waves crashing on the shores of faraway islands.

3 cups shredded carrots
1 cup (one 8-ounce can) canned crushed pineapple, drained and 2 tablespoons juice reserved
¼ cup raisins
¼ cup Kraft fat-free mayonnaise
Sugar substitute to equal 2 teaspoons sugar
¼ teaspoon coconut extract

In a large bowl, combine carrots, pineapple, and raisins. In a small bowl, combine mayonnaise, sugar substitute, reserved 2 tablespoons pineapple juice, and coconut extract. Add to carrot mixture. Mix gently to combine. Refrigerate at least 30 minutes. Gently stir again just before serving.

Each serving equals:

HE: 1½ Vegetable • 1 Fruit • 11 Optional Calories

133 Calories • 1 gm Fat • 1 gm Protein • 30 gm Carbohydrate • 143 mg Sodium • 2 gm Fiber

DIABETIC: 1½ Vegetable • 1 Fruit

Quick Spinach Salad

Serves 4 (1¼ cups)

I think Popeye would really approve of this easy and good-tasting spinach dish. And I'm sure Olive Oyl would appreciate its quick preparation!

4 cups torn fresh spinach, rinsed and stems removed
1 cup shredded carrots
1 cup thinly sliced radishes
1 tablespoon Hormel Bacon Bits
¼ cup Kraft fat-free Italian dressing

In a large bowl, combine spinach, carrots, radishes, and bacon bits. Add Italian dressing; toss gently to coat. Refrigerate at least 15 minutes. Toss again just before serving.

Each serving equals:

HE: 3 Vegetable • 12 Optional Calories

49 Calories • 1 gm Fat • 3 gm Protein • 7 gm Carbohydrate • 202 mg Sodium • 1 gm Fiber

DIABETIC: 2 Vegetable

Ranchero Vegetable Salad

Serves 8 (½ cup)

Even Cliff, who has sworn off anything with broccoli in it, reluctantly gave this a try and then promptly licked his plate clean. I think because of all the flavors mingling in this colorful salad, the broccoli sort of loses its distinct personality.

2 cups fresh broccoli florets
1¾ cups shredded carrots
¼ cup chopped red onion
¾ cup (3 ounces) shredded Kraft reduced-fat Cheddar cheese
¾ cup Kraft fat-free Catalina dressing
1 teaspoon chili seasoning mix

In a medium bowl, combine broccoli, carrots, red onion, and Cheddar cheese. Add dressing and chili seasoning. Mix gently to combine. Cover and refrigerate at least 30 minutes.

Each serving equals:

HE: 1 Vegetable • ½ Protein • ¼ Slider • 7 Optional Calories

78 Calories • 2 gm Fat • 4 gm Protein • 11 gm Carbohydrate • 267 mg Sodium • 1 gm Fiber

DIABETIC: 2 Vegetable • ½ Meat

Salsa Zucchini Salad

Serves 6 (⅔ cup)

Even if you're convinced you don't like zucchini, please don't pass on this recipe until you give it a try. I think you will be pleasantly surprised. My son Tommy has said more than once that he could live forever without ever eating zucchini. But all I can tell you is that he asked for seconds on this salad.

1 cup chunky salsa
⅓ cup Kraft fat-free Ranch dressing
¼ cup Kraft fat-free mayonnaise
1 teaspoon dried parsley flakes
3 cups diced zucchini

In a medium bowl, combine salsa, Ranch dressing, mayonnaise, and parsley flakes. Stir in zucchini. Mix well to combine. Cover and refrigerate at least 1 hour. Gently stir again just before serving.

Each serving equals:

HE: 1⅓ Vegetable • ¼ Slider • 3 Optional Calories

44 Calories • 0 gm Fat • 1 gm Protein • 10 gm Carbohydrate • 355 mg Sodium • 1 gm Fiber

DIABETIC: 2 Vegetable

Shrimp Caesar Salad

Serves 4 (2 cups)

Notice what I'm using for croutons in this "show-stopping" main dish salad? Who says cereal must only be eaten at breakfast time?

6 cups torn Romaine lettuce
4 ounces frozen or canned shrimp, rinsed and drained
¾ cup (3 ounces) shredded Kraft reduced-fat mozzarella cheese
1 scant cup (¾ ounce) Rice Chex
¼ cup (¾ ounce) grated Kraft House Italian or *Parmesan cheese*
⅓ cup Kraft fat-free Ranch dressing
½ teaspoon minced garlic
1 teaspoon lemon juice
½ teaspoon lemon pepper

In a large bowl, combine Romaine lettuce, shrimp, mozzarella cheese, and Rice Chex. Add House Italian cheese. Toss gently to combine. Refrigerate until ready to serve. Just before serving, in a small bowl, combine Ranch dressing, garlic, lemon juice, and lemon pepper. Add to Romaine lettuce mixture. Toss gently to combine. Serve at once.

Each serving equals:

HE: 3 Vegetable • 1¾ Protein • ¼ Bread • ¼ Slider • 11 Optional Calories

161 Calories • 5 gm Fat • 16 gm Protein • 13 gm Carbohydrate • 485 mg Sodium • 2 gm Fiber

DIABETIC: 2 Meat • ½ Starch • 1 Free Vegetable

Spinach Salad

Serves 4 (1⅓ cups)

I don't really care for cooked spinach, but I sure do love it fresh in a satisfying salad. If you share my sentiments, then I think you will be very pleased with my version of this traditional favorite.

4 cups fresh torn spinach
1 hard-boiled egg, chopped
2 tablespoons Hormel Bacon Bits
1 cup fresh sliced mushrooms
½ cup Kraft fat-free French dressing
1 tablespoon finely chopped onion
½ teaspoon Worcestershire sauce
1 tablespoon Brown Sugar Twin

In a medium bowl, combine spinach, chopped egg, bacon bits, and mushrooms. Refrigerate until ready to serve. Just before serving, in a small bowl, combine French dressing, onion, Worcestershire sauce, and Brown Sugar Twin. Add to spinach mixture. Toss well to coat. Serve at once.

Each serving equals:

HE: 2½ Vegetable • ¼ Protein (limited) • ½ Slider • 13 Optional Calories

90 Calories • 2 gm Fat • 5 gm Protein • 13 gm Carbohydrate • 267 mg Sodium • 1 gm Fiber

DIABETIC: 2 Vegetable • ½ Meat

Taffy Apple Salad

Serves 8 (full ⅔ cup)

I love making over high-calorie family favorites. This stupendous salad (some of you may consider this a dessert) was born when a friend asked me to redo a recipe that had been in her family for years. I threw out most of the traditional ingredients but managed to stir in the same flavor of the original.

1 (4-serving) package Jell-O sugar-free cook-and-serve vanilla pudding mix
1 (4-serving) package Jell-O sugar-free Hawaiian pineapple gelatin
1 cup water
1 tablespoon apple cider vinegar
2 cups diced unpeeled red apples (4 small)
1 cup (one 8-ounce can) canned crushed pineapple, packed in its own juice, drained
½ cup (2 ounces) chopped walnuts
¾ cup Yoplait plain fat-free yogurt
⅓ cup Carnation nonfat dry milk powder
Sugar substitute to equal ½ cup sugar
1 teaspoon vanilla extract
¾ cup Cool Whip Lite

In a small saucepan, combine dry pudding mix, dry gelatin, water, and vinegar. Bring mixture to a boil, stirring constantly. Remove from heat and refrigerate until cool, about 30 minutes. In a large bowl, combine diced apples, pineapple, and walnuts. Stir in cooled pudding mixture. In a medium bowl, combine yogurt and dry milk powder. Add sugar substitute and vanilla extract. Fold in Cool Whip Lite. Fold yogurt mixture into pudding mixture. Refrigerate at least 30 minutes. Gently stir again just before serving.

Each serving equals:

HE: ¾ Fruit • ½ Fat • ¼ Protein • ¼ Skim Milk • ¼ Slider • 9 Optional Calories

137 Calories • 5 gm Fat • 4 gm Protein • 19 gm Carbohydrate • 123 mg Sodium • 1 gm Fiber

DIABETIC: 1 Fruit • 1 Fat • ½ Starch

Tomato, Celery, and Cabbage Salad

Serves 4 (⅔ cup)

I always find that when my taste buds get a real "crunch" workout, I feel satisfied. See if you don't agree after taking one bite of this eye-catching bowl of veggies!

1 cup diced fresh tomatoes
1 cup chopped celery
1 cup chopped cabbage
1 hard-boiled egg, chopped
1 tablespoon Hormel Bacon Bits
¼ cup Kraft fat-free French dressing
1 tablespoon Kraft fat-free mayonnaise
1 teaspoon dried parsley flakes

In a medium bowl, combine tomatoes, celery, cabbage, egg, and bacon bits. Add French dressing, mayonnaise, and parsley flakes. Toss gently to combine. Cover and refrigerate at least 30 minutes. Gently stir again just before serving.

Each serving equals:

HE: 1½ Vegetable • ¼ Protein (limited) • ¼ Fat • 6 Optional Calories

66 Calories • 2 gm Fat • 3 gm Protein • 9 gm Carbohydrate • 203 mg Sodium • 1 gm Fiber

DIABETIC: 2 Vegetable

Vegetable Hodgepodge Salad

Serves 8 (1 cup)

If you've stayed away from vegetable salads because you thought one tasted just like the next, have I got a bowl of lip-smacking vitamins waiting for you!

1 cup diced zucchini
2 cups diced fresh tomatoes
1 cup diced green bell pepper
1 cup diced onion
1 cup finely chopped red radish
1 cup thinly sliced carrots
1 cup thinly sliced celery
½ cup Kraft fat-free French dressing
¼ cup Kraft fat-free Italian dressing
1 tablespoon chopped fresh parsley

In a large bowl, combine zucchini, tomatoes, green pepper, onion, radish, carrots, and celery. In a small bowl, combine French dressing, Italian dressing, and parsley. Pour dressing mixture over vegetables. Mix gently to combine. Cover and refrigerate at least 30 minutes. Gently stir again just before serving.

Each serving equals:

HE: 2 Vegetable • ¼ Slider • 2 Optional Calories

52 Calories • 0 gm Fat • 1 gm Protein • 12 gm Carbohydrate • 284 mg Sodium • 2 gm Fiber

DIABETIC: 2 Vegetable

Note: This is a bonus recipe, not included in any of the week's menus. But I had to include just one more way to stir up a vegetable salad. Just like your mother, I'm telling you to "eat your veggies, they're good for you!"

Vegetables

Breezy Green Beans

Cauliflower and Tomato au Gratin

Corn-Zucchini Sauté

Creamy Mashed Potatoes

Deviled Carrots

Grande Green Beans

Italian Copper Pennies

Mediterranean Tomatoes

Twice-Baked Potatoes

Wimp's Fresh Salsa

Breezy Green Beans

Serves 8 (⅔ cup)

This bean dish is such a breeze to prepare, but it will taste as if it took hours—and not a bit like "diet" food!

6 cups (three 16-ounce cans) canned French-style green beans, rinsed and drained
1 (8-ounce) package Philadelphia fat-free cream cheese
¼ teaspoon lemon pepper

In a large saucepan, combine beans, cream cheese, and lemon pepper. Heat over medium heat until cream cheese melts, stirring often. Serve at once.

Each serving equals:

HE: 1½ Vegetable • ½ Protein

44 Calories • 0 gm Fat • 5 gm Protein • 6 gm Carbohydrate • 257 mg Sodium • 1 gm Fiber

DIABETIC: 1 Vegetable • ½ Meat

Cauliflower and Tomato au Gratin

Serves 6 (¾ cup)

I think this very appealing dish provides a perfect marriage of flavors. The tomato sauce brings out the best in the cauliflower, and isn't that the idea behind all good relationships?

½ cup chopped onion
½ cup chopped green bell pepper
1¾ cups (one 15-ounce can) Hunt's Chunky Tomato Sauce
1 tablespoon Sprinkle Sweet or *Sugar Twin*
¼ teaspoon black pepper
1 teaspoon dried parsley flakes
¾ cup (3 ounces) Kraft shredded reduced-fat Cheddar cheese
3 cups cooked, chopped cauliflower
6 tablespoons (1½ ounces) dried fine bread crumbs

Preheat oven to 350 degrees. In a large skillet sprayed with butter-flavored cooking spray, sauté onion and green pepper until tender, about 5 minutes. Stir in tomato sauce, Sprinkle Sweet, black pepper, and parsley flakes. Add Cheddar cheese. Mix well to combine. Continue cooking, stirring often, until cheese melts. Stir in cauliflower. Pour mixture into an 8-by-8-inch baking dish sprayed with butter-flavored cooking spray. Evenly sprinkle bread crumbs over top. Bake 25 to 30 minutes. Place baking dish on a wire rack and let set 5 minutes. Cut into 6 pieces.

Each serving equals:

HE: 2½ Vegetable • ⅔ Protein • ⅓ Bread • 1 Optional Calorie

102 Calories • 2 gm Fat • 7 gm Protein • 14 gm Carbohydrate • 654 mg Sodium • 2 gm Fiber

DIABETIC: 2 Vegetable • ½ Meat • ½ Starch

Corn-Zucchini Sauté

Serves 4 (¾ cup)

If neither you nor your friends have a garden full of zucchini, don't despair! Just "pick" your own at the local farmers' market or produce stand and celebrate the tastes of summer in this colorful and tasty sauté.

¼ cup Kraft fat-free Italian dressing
½ cup chopped green bell pepper
2 cups sliced zucchini
¼ cup chopped onion
2 cups frozen whole-kernel corn
¼ cup canned chopped pimiento

In a large skillet, heat Italian dressing. Add green pepper, zucchini, and onion. Cook over medium heat until vegetables are crisp-tender, about 5 minutes. Add corn and pimiento. Continue cooking until mixture is heated through, about 3 minutes, stirring often.

Each serving equals:

HE: 1½ Vegetable • 1 Bread • 4 Optional Calories

100 Calories • 0 gm Fat • 3 gm Protein • 22 gm Carbohydrate • 148 mg Sodium • 3 gm Fiber

DIABETIC: 1 Vegetable • 1 Starch

Creamy Mashed Potatoes

Serves 4 (½ cup)

My Irish heritage won't allow me to share any recipe for potatoes that wouldn't pass muster with my ancestors. Even if the ingredients used in my tummy-pleasing dish wouldn't have been found in the "auld sod" when Grandma Margaret Carey McAndrews made her voyage over to America, I still think she would approve of the dish's great flavor.

1½ cups water
1⅓ cups (3 ounces) instant potato flakes
⅓ cup Carnation nonfat dry milk powder
¾ cup Yoplait plain fat-free yogurt
1 tablespoon dried onion flakes
1 teaspoon dried parsley flakes
1 teaspoon prepared horseradish

In a medium saucepan, bring water to a boil. Remove from heat. Stir in dry potato flakes and dry milk powder. Add yogurt, onion flakes, parsley flakes, and horseradish. Mix gently to combine. Serve at once *or* cover until ready to serve.

Each serving equals:

HE: 1 Bread • ½ Skim Milk • 4 Optional Calories

120 Calories • 0 gm Fat • 6 gm Protein • 24 gm Carbohydrate • 79 mg Sodium • 1 gm Fiber

DIABETIC: 1 Starch • ½ Skim Milk

Deviled Carrots

Serves 4 (1 cup)

Be an angel—and serve this easy side dish to your family tonight. They just may think they are in heaven!

3 cups shredded carrots
½ cup chopped onion
¼ cup water
2 tablespoons Brown Sugar Twin
1 teaspoon prepared mustard
¼ teaspoon black pepper

In a large skillet sprayed with butter-flavored cooking spray, sauté carrots and onion for 5 minutes, stirring often. Add water. Lower heat. Cover and simmer 10 minutes, stirring occasionally. Stir in Brown Sugar Twin, mustard, and black pepper. Continue cooking 2 to 3 minutes, stirring often. Serve at once *or* cover until ready to serve.

Each serving equals:
HE: 1¾ Vegetable • 3 Optional Calories

48 Calories • 0 gm Fat • 1 gm Protein • 11 gm Carbohydrate • 47 mg Sodium • 2 gm Fiber

DIABETIC: 2 Vegetable

Grande Green Beans

Serves 4 (1¼ cups) ❄

After just one bite, you will see why I called this simple—but simply delicious—bean dish Grande!

½ cup chopped onion
3 cups frozen French-style green beans
⅛ teaspoon lemon pepper
½ cup (one 2.5-ounce jar) canned sliced mushrooms, drained
⅓ cup (1½ ounces) shredded Kraft reduced-fat Monterey Jack or *Cheddar cheese*

In a medium saucepan sprayed with butter-flavored cooking spray, cook onion until tender. Add beans and lemon pepper. Cover. Cook, stirring occasionally, until beans are thawed and separated, about 10 minutes. Remove cover. Add mushrooms; continue cooking, stirring occasionally until beans are just tender, about 5 minutes. Sprinkle with cheese. Cover and let stand 1 minute before serving.

Each serving equals:
HE: 2 Vegetable • ½ Protein

66 Calories • 2 gm Fat • 5 gm Protein • 7 gm Carbohydrate • 381 mg Sodium • 1 gm Fiber

DIABETIC: 2 Vegetable

Italian Copper Pennies

Serves 8 (full ½ cup)

If you have ever enjoyed the traditional carrot salad fondly called Copper Pennies at any family potluck, then you are going to love this healthy Italian version I created.

4 cups (two 16-ounce cans) canned carrots, rinsed and drained
½ cup finely chopped onion
½ cup chopped green bell pepper
1 (10¾-ounce) can Campbell's Healthy Request Tomato Soup
2 tablespoons Sprinkle Sweet or *Sugar Twin*
½ cup Kraft fat-free Italian dressing
¼ cup cider vinegar
2 teaspoons prepared mustard
2 teaspoons Worcestershire sauce

In a medium bowl, combine carrots, onion, and green pepper. In a small saucepan, combine tomato soup, Sprinkle Sweet, Italian dressing, vinegar, mustard, and Worcestershire sauce. Bring mixture to a boil. Remove from heat. Pour hot mixture over carrot mixture. Stir gently to combine. Cover and refrigerate at least 4 hours.

Each serving equals:
HE: 1¼ Vegetable • ½ Slider

---

65 Calories • 1 gm Fat • 1 gm Protein • 13 gm Carbohydrate • 301 mg Sodium • 1 gm Fiber

---

DIABETIC: 2 Vegetable

Mediterranean Tomatoes

Serves 4 (¾ cup)

Only four ingredients, but oh, the flavor! The feta cheese is the star of this attractive dish, which will make you dream of lying on a beach in sunny Greece!

2½ cups diced fresh tomatoes
½ cup chopped green bell pepper
3 tablespoons (¾ ounce) shredded reduced-fat feta cheese
2 tablespoons Kraft fat-free Italian dressing

In a medium bowl, combine tomatoes, green pepper, and cheese. Add Italian dressing. Mix gently to combine. Cover and refrigerate at least 30 minutes or until ready to serve. Gently stir again just before serving.

Each serving equals:
HE: 1½ Vegetable • ¼ Protein • 2 Optional Calories

---

33 Calories • 2 gm Fat • 1 gm Protein • 5 gm Carbohydrate • 137 mg Sodium • 1 gm Fiber

---

DIABETIC: 1 Vegetable • ½ Fat

Twice-Baked Potatoes

Serves 4

Here's a virtually fat-free version of a traditional and much-loved high-fat potato dish. Isn't it great that we can still enjoy the flavor of our favorite dishes once they graduate from "reform school"?

4 (5-ounce) baking potatoes
¾ cup Yoplait plain fat-free yogurt
⅓ cup Carnation nonfat dry milk powder
¼ cup (¾ ounce) grated Kraft House Italian or *Parmesan cheese*
1 tablespoon dried parsley flakes
⅛ teaspoon black pepper
Dash paprika

Preheat oven to 400 degrees. Wash potatoes and place them on a baking sheet. Bake about 1 hour or until potatoes are tender. Cut a thin lengthwise slice from the top of each potato. Scoop out potato pulp, leaving a thin shell. In a medium bowl, mash potato pulp until fluffy. In a small bowl, combine yogurt and dry milk powder. Add yogurt mixture to potato. Mix until well combined. Stir in cheese, parsley flakes, and black pepper. Evenly fill potato shells with potato mixture. Lightly sprinkle paprika over tops. Bake 20 minutes or until tops are lightly browned.

Each serving equals:
HE: 1 Bread • ½ Skim Milk • ¼ Protein

220 Calories • 1 gm Fat • 10 gm Protein • 43 gm Carbohydrate • 160 mg Sodium • 1 gm Fiber

DIABETIC: 2 Starch • ½ Skim Milk • ½ Meat

Wimp's Fresh Salsa

Serves 6 (⅔ cup)

This salsa is for everyone like me who enjoys the flavorful combination of veggies, but without smoke coming out of our ears! If you are like Cliff and love salsa on the hot side, just throw in a few jalapeño peppers.

4½ cups peeled and finely chopped fresh tomatoes
½ cup finely chopped onion
½ cup finely chopped celery
½ cup finely chopped green bell pepper
2 tablespoons white vinegar
½ teaspoon salt
Sugar substitute to equal 1 tablespoon sugar
1 teaspoon chili seasoning mix
¼ teaspoon black pepper

In a large bowl, combine tomatoes, onion, celery, and green bell pepper. Add vinegar, salt, sugar substitute, chili seasoning mix, and black pepper. Mix well to combine. Cover and refrigerate several hours or overnight.

Each serving equals:
HE: 2 Vegetable • 1 Optional Calorie

40 Calories • 0 gm Fat • 1 gm Protein • 9 gm Carbohydrate • 204 mg Sodium • 2 gm Fiber

DIABETIC: 2 Vegetable

Main Dishes

Bubble Pizza

Chicken Breasts with Raspberry Sauce

Chicken Taco Salad

Chili Kolaches

Easy "Lasagna" Casserole

Easy Veggie-Ham Dish

Fish Creole

Grandma's Salmon Loaf

Hawaiian Chicken Salad

Italian Loose Meat Sandwiches

Linguine with Tuna and Peas

Macaroni and Cheese with Tomatoes

Mexican Scalloped Potatoes

Norwegian Burgers with Mushroom Sauce

Sweet 'n' Sour Pork

Tuna-Cheddar Sandwiches

Tuna-Macaroni Stuffed Tomatoes

Waldorf Chicken Salad Pitas

Bubble Pizza

Serves 6

This fabulous pizza recipe can be ready so fast, you'll never need to call for home delivery again! After preparing this just once, I wonder if you'll ever go back to the traditional way—it's *that* good. (Hint—you just might want to buy stock in refrigerated biscuits *before* word of this recipe hits the streets.)

8 ounces ground 90% lean turkey or beef
1 (7.5-ounce) can Pillsbury refrigerated buttermilk biscuits
1 teaspoon pizza or *Italian seasoning*
1 teaspoon Sprinkle Sweet or *Sugar Twin*
1¾ cups (one 15-ounce can) Hunt's Chunky Tomato Sauce
1 cup (4 ounces) Kraft shredded reduced-fat mozzarella cheese

Preheat oven to 400 degrees. In a large skillet sprayed with olive-flavored cooking spray, brown meat. Meanwhile, cut biscuits into quarters. Evenly place biscuit pieces in a 10-inch deep-dish pie plate sprayed with olive-flavored cooking spray. Stir pizza seasoning and Sprinkle Sweet into tomato sauce. Evenly spoon sauce over biscuit pieces. Arrange browned meat over sauce. Sprinkle top with mozzarella cheese. Bake for 12 to 15 minutes or until biscuits are done. Place pie plate on a wire rack and let set 5 minutes before serving. Cut into 6 pieces.

Each serving equals:
HE: 1⅔ Protein • 1¼ Bread • ⅔ Vegetable

203 Calories • 7 gm Fat • 15 gm Protein • 20 gm Carbohydrate • 782 mg Sodium • 2 gm Fiber

DIABETIC: 2 Meat • 1 Starch • 1 Vegetable

Chicken Breasts with Raspberry Sauce

Serves 4 ❄

If you want to impress anyone with your culinary skills but don't want to spend hours in the kitchen with preparation and cleanup, then may I suggest this simple but elegant chicken entree? It may be the first time you've cooked a main dish flavored with such unusual ingredients, but I bet it won't be the last!

2 teaspoons reduced-calorie margarine
16 ounces skinless and boneless chicken breast, cut into 4 pieces
½ cup Diet Mountain Dew ☆
¼ cup raspberry spreadable fruit spread

In a large skillet, melt margarine. Place chicken pieces in skillet. Brown chicken on both sides. Lower heat. Reserve 1 tablespoon Diet Mountain Dew. Pour remaining Diet Mountain Dew over chicken. Cover and simmer 15 minutes or until chicken is tender. In a small bowl, combine remaining 1 tablespoon Diet Mountain Dew and raspberry spreadable fruit spread. Evenly drizzle over chicken pieces. Continue cooking 1 to 2 minutes or until sauce is warmed. When serving, place one piece of chicken on each plate and evenly drizzle any remaining sauce over top.

Each serving equals:
HE: 3 Protein • 1 Fruit • ¼ Fat

170 Calories • 2 gm Fat • 26 gm Protein • 12 gm Carbohydrate • 88 mg Sodium • 1 gm Fiber

DIABETIC: 3 Meat • 1 Fruit

Chicken Taco Salad

Serves 6

Olé Olé Olé! This taco salad still delivers all the traditional flavors, but the chicken offers a lighter version of this spicy and satisfying dish!

¾ cup chopped onion
1½ cups (8 ounces) diced cooked chicken breast
5 ounces (one 8-ounce can) canned pinto beans, rinsed and drained
½ cup water
1½ teaspoons taco seasoning
4 cups shredded lettuce
2 cups chopped fresh tomato
½ cup chopped green bell pepper
¾ cup (3 ounces) Kraft shredded reduced-fat Cheddar cheese
1½ cups (1½ ounces) Corn Chex
¾ cup chunky salsa
6 tablespoons Land O Lakes fat-free sour cream

In a large saucepan sprayed with olive-flavored cooking spray, brown onion. Stir in chicken, pinto beans, water, and taco seasoning. Mix well to combine. Lower heat. Simmer 10 minutes, stirring occasionally. Meanwhile, in a large serving bowl, combine lettuce, tomato, and green pepper. Spoon hot chicken mixture over lettuce mixture. Top with Cheddar cheese and Corn Chex. Toss gently to combine. For each serving, place about 2 cups mixture on a plate and top with 2 tablespoons salsa and 1 tablespoon sour cream.

Each serving equals:
HE: 3 Protein • 2⅔ Vegetables • ⅓ Bread • 15 Optional Calories

232 Calories • 4 gm Fat • 22 gm Protein • 27 gm Carbohydrate • 344 mg Sodium • 5 gm Fiber

DIABETIC: 2 Meat • 2 Vegetable • 1 Starch

HINT: If you don't have leftovers, purchase a chunk of chicken breast from your local deli.

Chili Kolaches

Serves 8 (2 each) ❄

What isn't Irish in me is Bohemian. My Grandma Nowachek might wonder about these Mexican main-dish rolls inspired by her kolaches, but I'm sure after she tried one she would be pleased. My son Tommy thought they were wonderful. And this is coming from the kid who told me when he was six that he was "allergic" to pinto and kidney beans!

16 frozen yeast dinner rolls
10 ounces (one 16-ounce can) canned pinto beans, rinsed and drained
1 cup chunky salsa
1 teaspoon chili seasoning mix
½ cup plus 1 tablespoon (2¼ ounces) shredded Kraft reduced-fat Cheddar cheese

Preheat oven to 400 degrees. Spray a large cookie sheet with olive-flavored cooking spray. Evenly space frozen rolls on sheet. Cover with cloth and let thaw and rise, about 4 hours. Make an indentation in center of each roll. In a medium bowl, mash pinto beans with a fork. Add salsa, chili seasoning mix, and Cheddar cheese. Place full tablespoon of mixture in center of each roll. Cover loosely again with cloth and let rolls rest for 10 minutes. Quickly spray top of each roll with olive-flavored cooking spray. Bake 12 to 15 minutes or until golden brown. Remove from oven and quickly spray again with olive-flavored cooking spray. Good warm or cold.

Each serving equals:
HE: 2 Bread • 1 Protein

223 Calories • 3 gm Fat • 11 gm Protein • 38 gm Carbohydrate • 379 mg Sodium • 3 gm Fiber

DIABETIC: 2 Starch • 1 Meat

Easy "Lasagna" Casserole

Serves 4

My daughter-in-law, Pam, loves a good lasagna. She doesn't care if it is easy or healthy as long as it tastes the way *real* lasagna should taste. She gladly gives my quick casserole her seal of approval.

8 ounces ground 90% lean turkey or beef
½ cup finely chopped onion
1¾ cups (one 15-ounce can) Hunt's chunky tomato sauce
1 teaspoon Italian seasoning
⅔ cup Carnation nonfat dry milk powder
½ cup water
½ cup (4 ounces) Philadelphia fat-free cream cheese
¼ teaspoon minced garlic
1 teaspoon dried parsley flakes
2 cups cooked medium-width noodles
½ cup plus 1 tablespoon (2¼ ounces) shredded Kraft reduced-fat mozzarella cheese

Preheat oven to 375 degrees. In a large saucepan sprayed with olive-flavored cooking spray, brown meat and onion. Stir in tomato sauce and Italian seasoning. Lower heat and simmer 10 minutes. Meanwhile in a medium saucepan, combine dry milk powder, water, and cream cheese. Add garlic and parsley flakes. Cook over medium heat, stirring constantly, until cream cheese melts. Stir in cooked noodles. Pour noodle mixture into an 8-by-8-inch baking dish sprayed with olive-flavored cooking spray. Spread meat mixture evenly over noodle mixture. Evenly sprinkle mozzarella cheese over top. Bake, uncovered, 15 to 20 minutes. Let set 5 minutes before serving. Cut into 4 pieces.

Each serving equals:

HE: 2¾ Protein • 2 Vegetable • 1 Bread • ½ Skim Milk

---

328 Calories • 8 gm Fat • 28 gm Protein • 36 gm Carbohydrate • 773 mg Sodium • 2 gm Fiber

---

DIABETIC: 3 Meat • 2 Starch • 1 Vegetable

HINT: 1¾ cups uncooked noodles usually makes about 2 cups cooked.

Easy Veggie-Ham Dish

Serves 6

If you love ham, then why not enjoy what you love, now that it's available in delicious reduced-fat and reduced-sodium versions? Eating well for a lifetime means enjoying the healthiest possible version of your favorite dishes.

4 cups (one 16-ounce bag) frozen broccoli, cauliflower, and carrots
1 (10¾-ounce) can Campbell's Healthy Request Cream of Mushroom Soup
¾ cup (3 ounces) Kraft shredded reduced-fat Cheddar cheese
½ cup skim milk
1½ cups cooked rice
1 cup (6 ounces) finely diced Dubuque 97% fat-free ham or *any extra-lean ham*

Preheat oven to 350 degrees. In a medium saucepan, cook vegetables in water until crisp-tender, about 5 minutes. Drain. In same saucepan, combine mushroom soup, Cheddar cheese, and skim milk. Cook over medium heat, stirring often, until Cheddar cheese melts. Stir in rice, ham, and drained vegetables. Mix well to combine. Spread mixture into an 8-by-8-inch baking dish sprayed with butter-flavored cooking spray. Bake 25 to 30 minutes. Place baking dish on a wire rack and let set for 5 minutes. Cut into 6 pieces.

Each serving equals:
HE: 1⅓ Vegetable • 1⅓ Protein • ½ Bread • ¼ Slider • 17 Optional Calories

131 Calories • 3 gm Fat • 11 gm Protein • 15 gm Carbohydrate • 381 mg Sodium • 2 gm Fiber

DIABETIC: 1 Vegetable • 1 Meat • 1 Starch

HINT: 1. 1 cup uncooked rice usually yields about 1½ cups cooked.
2. 1½ cups broccoli, 1½ cups cauliflower, and 1 cup carrots (fresh or frozen) can be used instead of blended vegetables.

Fish Creole

Serves 4 (1 full cup fish mixture over ½ cup rice) ❄

If you think fish has to be steamed, poached, or oven baked to be healthy, think again. Then give this flavorful dish a try. My guess is it will become a mainstay among your favorite fish dishes.

½ cup chopped onion
½ cup chopped celery
½ cup chopped green bell pepper
1¾ cups (one 15-ounce can) Hunt's chunky tomato sauce
½ teaspoon minced garlic
1 teaspoon Worcestershire sauce
16 ounces white fish fillets, cut into 16 pieces
2 cups cooked rice

In a large skillet sprayed with butter-flavored cooking spray, sauté onion, celery, and green pepper until tender. Stir in tomato sauce, garlic, and Worcestershire sauce. Add fish pieces. Lower heat. Cover and simmer 20 minutes, stirring occasionally.

Each serving equals:
HE: 2½ Vegetable • 1½ Protein • 1 Bread

197 Calories • 1 gm Fat • 25 gm Protein • 22 gm Carbohydrate • 721 mg Sodium • 3 gm Fiber

DIABETIC: 3 Meat • 1½ Starch • 1 Vegetable

HINT: 1⅓ cups dry rice will usually make 2 cups cooked.

Grandma's Salmon Loaf

Serves 6

Here's one of those foods that recalls happy memories at the same time it delivers lots of good nutrition and flavor. This salmon loaf reminds me of the "old-time" salmon loaf my mother and grandmother used to make. I think it's the little bit of onion that gives it a special touch.

⅔ cup Carnation nonfat dry milk powder
1⅓ cups water
1 (14¾-ounce) can salmon with juice, flaked
¼ cup chopped onion
28 small fat-free saltine crackers, made into crumbs (2 cups)
1 egg or equivalent in egg substitute
¼ teaspoon lemon pepper

Preheat oven to 350 degrees. In a large bowl, combine dry milk powder and water. Add salmon, onion, crackers, egg, and lemon pepper. Mix well to combine. Let set 2 to 3 minutes for crackers to absorb moisture. Pat into a 9-by-5-inch loaf pan sprayed with butter-flavored cooking spray. Bake 40 to 45 minutes. Place baking dish on a wire rack and let set 5 minutes. Cut into 6 pieces.

Each serving equals:
HE: 2⅔ Protein • ⅔ Bread • ½ Skim Milk

183 Calories • 5 gm Fat • 18 gm Protein • 16 gm Carbohydrate • 545 mg Sodium • 1 gm Fiber

DIABETIC: 2 Meat • 1 Starch

Hawaiian Chicken Salad

Serves 4 (full 1½ cups)

This tasty salad is not only attractive to the eye, it's oh-so-filling too! Cooking the macaroni and frozen green beans together saves both time and dirty pots!

1 full cup (3 ounces) uncooked elbow macaroni
2 cups frozen green beans
1 cup water
1 full cup (6 ounces) diced cooked chicken breast
1 cup chopped celery
¼ cup slivered almonds (1 ounce)
1 cup (one 8-ounce can) canned pineapple chunks, packed in their own juice, drained and 1 tablespoon juice reserved
¾ cup Yoplait plain fat-free yogurt
⅓ cup Kraft fat-free mayonnaise

In a large saucepan, cook macaroni and green beans together in water until green beans are tender, about 15 minutes. Drain and rinse well. In a large bowl, combine diced chicken, celery, almonds, and pineapple. Stir in macaroni and green bean mixture. In a small bowl, combine yogurt, mayonnaise, and 1 tablespoon reserved pineapple juice. Add to chicken mixture. Cover and refrigerate at least 2 hours. Gently stir again just before serving.

Each serving equals:
HE: 1¾ Protein • 1½ Vegetable • 1 Bread • ½ Fruit • ½ Fat • ¼ Milk • 12 Optional Calories

298 Calories • 6 gm Fat • 21 gm Protein • 40 gm Carbohydrate • 201 mg Sodium • 2 gm Fiber

DIABETIC: 2 Starch • 1½ Meat • 1 Vegetable • ½ Fruit

Italian Loose Meat Sandwiches

Serves 6 (⅓ cup meat mixture) ❄

We have a tradition here in the Midwest of serving browned ground meat spooned loosely on buns and calling it a Loose Meat Sandwich. Well, I just took that tradition one step further by adding Italian seasoning and mushrooms. Viva la differenza!

16 ounces ground 90% lean turkey or beef
½ cup chopped onion
1 cup (one 8-ounce can) canned tomato sauce
½ cup (one 2.5-ounce jar) canned sliced mushrooms, drained
1 tablespoon Sprinkle Sweet or Sugar Twin
1 teaspoon Italian seasoning
6 reduced-calorie hamburger buns

In a large skillet sprayed with olive-flavored cooking spray, brown meat and onion. Add tomato sauce, mushrooms, Sprinkle Sweet, and Italian seasoning. Mix well to combine. Lower heat and simmer 10 to 15 minutes. Serve mixture on hamburger buns.

Each serving equals:

HE: 2 Protein • 1 Bread • 1 Vegetable • 1 Optional Calorie

203 Calories • 7 gm Fat • 16 gm Protein • 19 gm Carbohydrate • 467 mg Sodium • 2 gm Fiber

DIABETIC: 2 Meat • 1 Bread • ½ Vegetable

Linguine with Tuna and Peas

Serves 4 (1 cup) ❄

This is really just an updated version of tuna and noodles prepared on top of the stove instead of baked in the oven. The cheese adds just the right touch of tangy flavor.

1½ cups (one 12-fluid-ounce can) Carnation evaporated skim milk
3 tablespoons flour
¼ teaspoon black pepper
½ cup frozen peas
1 (6-ounce) can white albacore tuna, packed in water, drained and flaked
¼ cup (¾ ounce) grated Kraft House Italian or *Parmesan cheese*
2 cups cooked linguine

In a covered jar, combine evaporated skim milk and flour. Shake well. Pour mixture into a large skillet sprayed with butter-flavored cooking spray. Add black pepper and peas. Cook over medium heat, stirring constantly, until mixture thickens. Add tuna, cheese, and cooked linguine. Mix well to combine. Lower heat. Continue cooking, stirring constantly, about 5 minutes or until mixture is heated through.

Each serving equals:

HE: 1½ Bread • 1 Protein • ¾ Skim Milk

279 Calories • 3 gm Fat • 25 gm Protein • 38 gm Carbohydrate • 304 mg Sodium • 2 gm Fiber

DIABETIC: 2 Meat • 1 Skim Milk • 1 Starch

HINT: 1½ cups dry broken linguine usually makes 2 cups cooked.

Macaroni and Cheese with Tomatoes

Serves 4 ❄

I took two of my favorite "comfort foods" and made a new favorite.

½ cup chopped onion
1½ cups (one 12-fluid-ounce can) Carnation evaporated skim milk
3 tablespoons flour
1 full cup (4½ ounces) shredded Kraft reduced-fat Cheddar cheese
2½ cups cooked elbow macaroni
2 tablespoons Hormel Bacon Bits
2 cups (one 16-ounce can) canned tomatoes, drained and chopped
⅛ teaspoon black pepper
1 teaspoon parsley flakes

Preheat oven to 350 degrees. In a large skillet sprayed with butter-flavored cooking spray, sauté onion until tender. In a covered jar, combine evaporated skim milk and flour. Shake well. Pour milk mixture into skillet with onion. Stir in Cheddar cheese. Continue cooking, stirring constantly until sauce thickens and cheese melts. Add cooked macaroni, bacon bits, drained canned tomatoes, black pepper, and parsley flakes. Mix well to combine. Pour mixture into an 8-by-8-inch baking dish sprayed with butter-flavored cooking spray. Bake 15 minutes. Let set 5 minutes before serving. Cut into 4 pieces.

Each serving equals:

HE: 1½ Bread • 1½ Protein • 1¼ Vegetable • ¾ Skim Milk • 15 Optional Calories

359 Calories • 7 gm Fat • 25 gm Protein • 49 gm Carbohydrate • 537 mg Sodium • 2 gm Fiber

DIABETIC: 2 Starch • 1½ Meat • 1 Vegetable • 1 Skim Milk

HINT: 2 cups uncooked macaroni usually makes about 2½ cups cooked.

Mexican Scalloped Potatoes

Serves 4

This scalloped potatoes and ham dish with the South-of-the-Border flavor made a BIG impression on my "meat and potatoes" guy. Because each serving includes an entire cup of hash browns, you'll be delighted to discover how satisfying and filling this dish is!

4 cups (15 ounces) shredded potatoes or *purchased frozen hash browns, thawed* ☆
1 full cup (6 ounces) diced Dubuque 97% fat-free ham or *any extra-lean ham*
1½ cups (one 12-fluid-ounce can) Carnation evaporated skim milk
3 tablespoons flour
¾ cup chopped onion
1¾ cups (one 15-ounce can) Mexican stewed tomatoes, drained
¾ cup (3 ounces) shredded Kraft reduced-fat Cheddar cheese ☆
½ teaspoon chili seasoning mix

Preheat oven to 350 degrees. Place half of potatoes in bottom of an 8-by-8-inch baking dish. Layer with diced ham.

In a covered jar, combine milk and flour. Shake well. Spray a medium saucepan with butter-flavored cooking spray. Pour milk mixture into saucepan and cook over medium heat until mixture thickens, stirring constantly. Add onion, drained stewed tomatoes, ½ cup Cheddar cheese, and chili seasoning. Mix well to combine. Continue cooking until cheese melts. Pour half of mixture over potatoes and ham. Place remaining potatoes on top and pour rest of sauce mixture over potatoes. Sprinkle remaining Cheddar cheese on top. Bake 30 to 35 minutes. Let set 5 minutes before serving. Cut into 4 pieces.

Each serving equals:

HE: 2 Protein • 1 Vegetable • 1 Bread • ¾ Skim Milk

313 Calories • 5 gm Fat • 24 gm Protein • 43 gm Carbohydrate • 628 mg Sodium • 2 gm Fiber

DIABETIC: 2 Meat • 1½ Starch • 1 Vegetable • 1 Skim Milk

HINTS:
1. Mr. Dell's shredded potatoes are a good choice for this recipe.
2. If you can't find Mexican stewed tomatoes, use regular and 1 teaspoon Taco seasoning.

Norwegian Burgers with Mushroom Sauce

Serves 6 ❄

Since my last name is LUND, were you beginning to wonder if I was ever going to share a Norwegian dish? Cliff, my good-looking Norwegian husband, loved this wonderfully aromatic, palate-tempting dish. It's amazing how a small amount of nutmeg can make this otherwise almost ordinary dish really shine!

6 tablespoons (1½ ounces) dried fine bread crumbs
1 tablespoon dried onion flakes
1 teaspoon dried parsley flakes
¼ teaspoon nutmeg
16 ounces ground 90% lean turkey or beef
½ cup skim milk ☆
1 (10¾-ounce) can Campbell's Healthy Request Cream of Mushroom Soup

In a large bowl, combine bread crumbs, onion flakes, parsley flakes, and nutmeg. Add meat and ¼ cup skim milk. Mix well to combine. Using a ⅓-cup measuring cup as a guide, form into 6 patties. Place patties in a large skillet sprayed with butter-flavored cooking spray. Cover and cook over medium heat 7 to 8 minutes on each side. Transfer browned patties to a hot platter. In same skillet, combine mushroom soup and remaining ¼ cup skim milk. Cook over medium heat, stirring constantly, until mixture is heated through. Evenly spoon mushroom soup mixture over browned patties. Serve at once.

Each serving equals:

HE: 2 Protein • ⅓ Bread • ¼ Slider • 15 Optional Calories

163 Calories • 7 gm Fat • 15 gm Protein • 10 gm Carbohydrate • 347 mg Sodium • 0 gm Fiber

DIABETIC: 2 Meat • ½ Starch

Sweet 'n' Sour Pork

Serves 6 (1 cup)

My son James loves Chinese pork dishes, including this one I created with him in mind. He was somewhat surprised to learn, though, that the tangy sweet flavor came from spreadable fruit. Now he no longer considers fruit spread something to put only on toast.

16 ounces lean pork tenderloin, cut into thin strips
½ cup finely chopped onion
¼ cup vinegar
1 tablespoon cornstarch
¼ teaspoon ginger (optional)
⅛ teaspoon black pepper
¼ cup apricot spreadable fruit spread
1 cup green and/or red pepper, cut in strips
1 cup (one 8-ounce can) canned pineapple chunks, packed in their own juice, drained

In a large skillet sprayed with butter-flavored cooking spray, sauté pork about 5 minutes over medium heat. Add onion; lower heat. Cover and simmer 10 minutes. In a small bowl, combine vinegar, cornstarch, ginger, and black pepper. Add to mixture in skillet. Add spreadable fruit spread and pepper strips. Bring mixture to a boil, stirring constantly. Lower heat. Cover and simmer 5 minutes. Add pineapple chunks and heat through.

Each serving equals:
HE: 2 Protein • 1 Fruit • ½ Vegetable • 5 Optional Calories

---

200 Calories • 8 gm Fat • 19 gm Protein • 13 gm Carbohydrate • 209 mg Sodium • 1 gm Fiber

---

DIABETIC: 2 Meat • 1 Fruit

HINT: Good served with rice.

Tuna-Cheddar Sandwiches

Serves 4

You may never again be satisfied eating a plain tuna sandwich. The Cheddar cheese adds just the right rich texture and flavor.

1 (6-ounce) can tuna, packed in water, drained and flaked
⅓ cup (1½ ounces) shredded Kraft reduced-fat Cheddar cheese
¼ cup Kraft fat-free mayonnaise
1 tablespoon pickle relish
¼ teaspoon black pepper
8 slices reduced-calorie bread

In a medium bowl, combine tuna and Cheddar cheese. Add mayonnaise, pickle relish, and black pepper. Mix gently to combine. Spread about ¼ cup of mixture over 4 slices of bread. Top with remaining bread slices. Serve at once or refrigerate until ready to serve.

Each serving equals:
HE: 1¼ Protein • 1 Bread • 14 Optional Calories

---

170 Calories • 2 gm Fat • 20 gm Protein • 18 gm Carbohydrate • 378 mg Sodium • 1 gm Fiber

---

DIABETIC: 2 Meat • 1 Starch

Tuna-Macaroni Stuffed Tomatoes

Serves 4

Here's a great lunch idea for those steamy, too-hot-to-cook summer days. Well, you *will* have to boil the macaroni for this salad unless you have leftovers in the fridge. But it'll just take a few minutes to cook while you relax in the backyard or living room, sipping on a tall glass of my classic recipe for "Homemade" Limeade.

1 (6-ounce) can tuna, packed in water, drained and flaked
1½ cups cooked elbow macaroni
1 cup diced celery
2 teaspoons dried onion flakes
⅓ cup Kraft fat-free mayonnaise
2 tablespoons canned chopped pimiento
4 medium tomatoes

In a medium bowl, combine tuna, macaroni, celery, and onion flakes. Add mayonnaise and pimiento. Mix well to combine. Split each tomato into 4 wedges, but *do not* cut all the way to the bottom. Evenly stuff about ⅔ cup tuna mixture into each tomato. Refrigerate at least 30 minutes.

Each serving equals:

HE: 1½ Vegetable • ¾ Bread • ¾ Protein • 13 Optional Calories

161 Calories • 1 gm Fat • 7 gm Protein • 31 gm Carbohydrate • 164 mg Sodium • 5 gm Fiber

DIABETIC: 1½ Vegetable • 1 Starch • 1 Meat

HINT: 1 cup uncooked macaroni usually cooks to about 1½ cups.

Waldorf Chicken Salad Pitas

Serves 4

A satisfying sandwich to savor either at home, at school, or at the office. The filling is so good, it's almost worthy of being served at New York's Waldorf-Astoria Hotel!

1 cup (5 ounces) diced cooked chicken breast
1 cup diced red apples (2 small)
¼ cup raisins
½ cup diced celery
¼ cup (1 ounce) chopped walnuts
¼ cup Kraft fat-free mayonnaise
1 teaspoon lemon juice
2 pita rounds

In a medium bowl, combine chicken, apples, raisins, celery, and walnuts. Add mayonnaise and lemon juice. Mix well to combine. Cut pita rounds in half. Stuff full ½ cup of mixture into each pita half. Serve at once or refrigerate until ready to serve.

Each serving equals:

HE: 1½ Protein • 1 Bread • 1 Fruit • ½ Fat • ¼ Vegetable • 10 Optional Calories

254 Calories • 6 gm Fat • 15 gm Protein • 35 gm Carbohydrate • 297 mg Sodium • 2 gm Fiber

DIABETIC: 1½ Meat • 1 Starch • 1 Fruit

Desserts

Acapulco Gold Pudding

Almost Sinless Sundae Pie

Baked Apple

Cherry Kolaches

Dewy Mountain Strawberry Cheesecake

Dwayne's Coconut Banana Chocolate Cream Pie

Frozen Yogurt Tarts

Lemon Rice Pudding

Mexican Cinnamon Mocha Cake

Oatmeal Bars

Orange Pudding Treats

New England Pumpkin Raisin Pie

Raspberry Cream Tarts

S'Mores Pudding

Soda Fountain Delight

South Seas Chocolate Tarts

Wacky Spice Cake

Wonderful Butterscotch Treasure Pie

Acapulco Gold Pudding

Serves 4 ❄

The best desserts don't always have to be the most difficult! This "golden" pudding treat is a perfect example of an easy, healthy dessert that looks and tastes almost "too good."

1 (4-serving) package Jell-O sugar-free instant vanilla pudding mix
⅓ cup Carnation nonfat dry milk powder
1 cup (one 8-ounce can) canned crushed pineapple, packed in its own juice; undrained
¾ cup Yoplait plain fat-free yogurt
¼ cup (1 ounce) sliced almonds
2 tablespoons flaked coconut
Sugar substitute to equal 2 teaspoons sugar
Cinnamon
4 tablespoons Cool Whip Lite

In a medium bowl, combine dry pudding mix and dry milk powder. Add undrained pineapple and yogurt. Mix well using a wire whisk. Add almonds, coconut, and sugar substitute. Blend well. Spoon into 4 dessert dishes. Sprinkle dash of cinnamon on top of each. Refrigerate at least 30 minutes. Just before serving, top each with 1 tablespoon Cool Whip Lite.

Each serving equals:

HE: ½ Fruit • ½ Fat • ½ Skim Milk • ¼ Protein • ½ Slider • 1 Optional Calorie

173 Calories • 5 gm Fat • 6 gm Protein • 26 gm Carbohydrate • 314 mg Sodium • 1 gm Fiber

DIABETIC: 1 Fruit • 1 Fat • ½ Skim Milk

Almost Sinless Sundae Pie

Serves 8 ❄

A radio host challenged me on the air to make over the original recipe for this dessert. He said that he thought it was as sinful as any pie he had ever eaten and he was convinced there was no way to redeem it. His version clocked in at 466 calories and 30 grams of fat per serving. Mine is of course so much lower in calories and fat that it is almost *sinless!*

1 (4-serving) package Jell-O sugar-free chocolate cook-and-serve pudding mix
⅔ cup Carnation nonfat dry milk powder
1 cup water
1 teaspoon vanilla extract
½ cup (1 ounce) miniature marshmallows
1 (6-ounce) Keebler butter-flavored piecrust
2 cups fat-free and sugar-free vanilla ice cream, slightly softened
2 tablespoons (½ ounce) chopped pecans
½ cup Cool Whip Lite
4 maraschino cherries, halved

In a medium saucepan, combine dry pudding mix and dry milk powder. Add water. Mix well to combine. Cook over medium heat, stirring constantly until mixture thickens and comes to a boil. Remove from heat. Stir in vanilla extract and marshmallows. Mix well until mixture is smooth. Cool 10 minutes. Spoon ice cream into piecrust. Drizzle chocolate mixture evenly over ice cream. Sprinkle pecans over top. Evenly drop Cool Whip Lite by 1 tablespoon to form 8 mounds. Place ½ maraschino cherry in center of each mound. Freeze until firm, at least 4 hours. Let set at room temperature at least 15 minutes before serving. Cut into 8 pieces.

Each serving equals:

HE: ½ Bread • ¼ Skim Milk • ¼ Fat • 1¼ Slider • 7 Optional Calories

215 Calories • 7 gm Fat • 5 gm Protein • 33 gm Carbohydrate • 308 mg Sodium • 1 gm Fiber

DIABETIC: 2 Starch • 1 Fat

HINT: Wells Blue Bunny Nonfat Sugar-Free Dairy Dessert is wonderful!

Baked Apple

Serves 1

Have you ever eaten an apple for a snack and ended up feeling *hungrier* than before you started? I think it's because our taste buds just start to have fun and then we tell them the party's over! This easy way to eat that same apple never leaves you hungry. Could it be the warmth that does the trick?

½ cup sliced cooking apple (1 small)
1 tablespoon Cary's sugar-free maple syrup

Place apple slices in a microwavable dish. Drizzle maple syrup evenly over apple. Cover. Cook on HIGH in microwave 4 to 5 minutes or until apple is tender.

Each serving equals:

HE: 1 Fruit • 10 Optional Calories

72 Calories • 0 gm Fat • 0 gm Protein • 18 gm Carbohydrate • 20 mg Sodium • 1 gm Fiber

DIABETIC: 1 Fruit

HINT: If using a conventional oven, bake at 350 degrees for 20 minutes or until apple is tender.

Cherry Kolaches

Serves 12

One of my fondest childhood memories is of my mother and grandmother baking kolaches. (If you've never had one, I'd describe it as a kind of sweet roll, but better than any you've tried. . . .) When I finished experimenting with this recipe, my son James said they were "almost" as good as Grandma's. What a compliment for a recipe that's almost fat and sugar free!

12 frozen yeast dinner rolls
1 (4-serving) package Jell-O sugar-free vanilla cook-and-serve pudding mix
¾ cup water
2–3 drops red food coloring
1½ cups cherries, no sugar added (frozen, fresh, or canned)
¼ teaspoon almond extract

Spray a large cookie sheet with butter-flavored cooking spray. Evenly space frozen rolls on sheet. Cover with cloth, and let thaw and rise. Make an indentation in center of each roll. In a medium saucepan, combine dry pudding mix, water, food coloring, and cherries. Cook over medium heat until thickened and sauce comes to a boil. Remove from heat. Stir in almond extract. Place 1 large tablespoon of sauce in center of each roll. Cover again and let rolls rest for 10 to 15 minutes. Quickly spray top of each roll with butter-flavored cooking spray. Bake 10 to 15 minutes at 400 degrees or until golden brown. Remove from oven and quickly spray again with butter-flavored cooking spray. Place sheet on top of wire rack and let cool.

Each serving equals:

HE: 1 Bread • ¼ Fruit • 7 Optional Calories

96 Calories • 1 gm Fat • 3 gm Protein • 18 gm Carbohydrate • 149 mg Sodium • 1 gm Fiber

DIABETIC: 1 Starch

Dewy Mountain Strawberry Cheesecake

Serves 8 ❄

This recipe was conceived when a good friend brought me a large bowl of fresh-from-the-garden strawberries. While I was deciding what to make with them, my eyes spotted a bottle of Diet Mountain Dew. I quickly wondered if I could make a no-bake cheesecake with the "Diet Dew" as the liquid. And the answer is: YES! YES! YES!

1 (8-ounce) package Philadelphia fat-free cream cheese
1 (4-serving) package Jell-O sugar-free instant vanilla pudding mix
⅔ cup Carnation nonfat dry milk powder
1 cup Diet Mountain Dew
1 (6-ounce) Keebler butter-flavored piecrust
¾ cup Cool Whip Lite
4 cups sliced fresh strawberries ☆
¼ cup Sprinkle Sweet or *Sugar Twin*

In a medium bowl, stir cream cheese until soft. Add dry pudding mix, dry milk powder, and Diet Mountain Dew. Mix well with a wire whisk. Pour into piecrust. Evenly spread Cool Whip Lite over top. Refrigerate. In a medium bowl, mash 1 cup strawberries with a fork or potato masher. Stir in Sprinkle Sweet. Add remaining strawberries. Mix well to combine. Cover and refrigerate until ready to use. When serving, cut pie into 8 pieces and spoon about ⅓ cup strawberry mixture over each piece.

Each serving equals:

HE: ½ Bread • ½ Protein • ½ Fruit • ¼ Skim Milk • ¾ Slider • 18 Optional Calories

202 Calories • 6 gm Fat • 7 gm Protein • 30 gm Carbohydrate • 411 mg Sodium • 2 gm Fiber

DIABETIC: 1 Starch • 1 Fruit • ½ Fat • ½ Meat

Dwayne's Coconut Banana Chocolate Cream Pie

Serves 8 ❄

When I was asked to be a guest on a local program, Dwayne, the host, specifically told Cliff I was to bring a Coconut Banana Chocolate Cream Pie. He wanted to see if he could stump me. Well, he was more than a little disappointed that I had to think for fewer than 5 minutes to create this irresistible response to his "challenge." But he wasn't a bit disappointed in the flavor of this spectacular dessert. . . .

1 (6-ounce) Keebler chocolate-flavored piecrust
2 cups sliced bananas (2 medium)
1 (4-serving) package Jell-O sugar-free instant chocolate pudding mix
⅔ cup Carnation nonfat dry milk powder
1⅓ cups water
1 cup Cool Whip Lite ☆
1½ teaspoons coconut extract ☆
2 tablespoons flaked coconut

Layer sliced bananas in piecrust. In a medium bowl, combine dry pudding mix and dry milk powder. Add water. Mix well using a wire whisk. Blend in ¼ cup Cool Whip Lite and ¾ teaspoon coconut extract. Spread mixture evenly over bananas. Refrigerate while preparing topping. In a small bowl, combine remaining ¾ cup Cool Whip Lite and remaining ¾ teaspoon coconut extract. Spread mixture evenly over set pudding mixture. Evenly sprinkle coconut over top. Refrigerate at least 2 hours. Cut into 8 pieces.

Each serving equals:

HE: ½ Bread • ½ Fruit • ¼ Skim Milk • 1 Slider • 2 Optional Calories

---

207 Calories • 7 gm Fat • 4 gm Protein • 32 gm Carbohydrate • 294 mg Sodium • 2 gm Fiber

---

DIABETIC: 1 Starch • 1 Fruit • 1 Fat

Frozen Yogurt Tarts

Serves 6 ❄

Why not let the kids help you make these ultra-easy desserts so they can impress Daddy and the grandparents with their budding culinary skills? Besides, after licking the bowl, they may never turn their noses up at yogurt again.

6 Keebler single-serve graham cracker shells
1 cup + 2 tablespoons Yoplait plain fat-free yogurt
6 tablespoons apricot spreadable fruit spread
¾ cup Cool Whip Lite
¼ teaspoon almond extract

In a medium bowl, combine yogurt and spreadable fruit spread. Blend in Cool Whip Lite and almond extract. Spoon mixture evenly into graham cracker shells. Place in freezer and freeze until firm, at least 2 hours. Remove from freezer 15 minutes before serving.

Each serving equals:

HE: 1 Fruit • ½ Bread • ⅓ Skim Milk • ¾ Slider • 6 Optional Calories

---

186 Calories • 6 gm Fat • 3 gm Protein • 30 gm Carbohydrate • 167 mg Sodium • 2 gm Fiber

---

DIABETIC: 1 Starch • 1 Fruit • 1 Fat

Lemon Rice Pudding

Serves 6 (¾ cup) ❄

Once I figured out how to make sugar-free instant lemon pudding using ingredients found in my small town, I had a HEYDAY coming up with new recipes. This is one at the top of my list. Of course, I combined my two favorites (lemon pudding and rice pudding) for this palate-pleasing pleasure.

1 (4-serving) package Jell-O sugar-free instant vanilla pudding mix
1 (4-serving) package Jell-O sugar-free lemon gelatin
⅔ cup Carnation nonfat dry milk powder
1¾ cups water
½ cup Cool Whip Lite
3 cups cooked rice

In a large bowl, combine dry pudding mix, dry gelatin, and dry milk powder. Add water. Mix well using a wire whisk. Blend in Cool Whip Lite. Add cooked rice, mixing gently to combine. Evenly spoon mixture into 6 dessert dishes. Refrigerate at least 10 minutes.

Each serving equals:

HE: 1 Bread • ⅓ Skim Milk • ¼ Slider • 13 Optional Calories

---

137 Calories • 1 gm Fat • 5 gm Protein • 27 gm Carbohydrate • 253 mg Sodium • 1 gm Fiber

---

DIABETIC: 2 Starch

HINT: 2¼ cups dry rice usually makes 3 cups cooked

Mexican Cinnamon Mocha Cake

Serves 12

I served this "melt-in-your-mouth" confectionery delight to my sisters, Mary and Regina. Both just shook their heads and kept wondering how anything that used fat-free mayo as the "fat" could taste so good.

1½ cups flour
¼ cup unsweetened cocoa
1 cup Carnation nonfat dry milk powder ☆
1¼ teaspoons baking soda
½ cup Sprinkle Sweet or *Sugar Twin*
1½ teaspoons cinnamon ☆
1½ teaspoons dry coffee crystals ☆
¾ cup Kraft fat-free mayonnaise
2 cups water ☆
1 teaspoon chocolate extract
1½ teaspoons vanilla extract ☆
1 (4-serving) package Jell-O sugar-free instant chocolate fudge pudding mix
½ cup Cool Whip Lite

Preheat oven to 350 degrees. In a large bowl, combine flour, cocoa, ⅓ cup dry milk powder, baking soda, Sprinkle Sweet, 1 teaspoon cinnamon, and 1 teaspoon dry coffee crystals. In another bowl, combine mayonnaise, 1 cup water, chocolate extract, and 1 teaspoon vanilla extract. Mix well to combine. Add mayonnaise mixture to flour mixture. Mix well just to combine. Pour mixture into a 9-by-9-inch cake pan sprayed with butter-flavored cooking spray. Bake 18 to 22 minutes or until cake tests done in center. Place pan on wire rack and cool for 45 minutes. In a medium bowl, combine dry pudding mix, remaining ⅔ cup dry milk powder, remaining ½ teaspoon cinnamon, and remaining ½ teaspoon coffee crystals. Mix well to combine. Add remaining 1 cup water and remaining ½ teaspoon vanilla extract. Mix well using a wire whisk. Blend in Cool Whip Lite.

Spread pudding mixture evenly over cooled cake. Cut into 12 pieces. Refrigerate leftovers.

Each serving equals:

HE: ⅔ Bread • ¼ Skim Milk • ½ Slider • 11 Optional Calories

114 Calories • 1 gm Fat • 4 gm Protein • 22 gm Carbohydrate • 376 mg Sodium • 1 gm Fiber

DIABETIC: 1½ Starch

Note: Here's another bonus recipe. It is not included in the week's menus. But every healthy cook needs a delicious, good-for-you celebration cake. Enjoy!

Oatmeal Bars

Serves 8 (2 bars)

These hearty treats usually put a smile on the face of any man I've served them to. My grandsons, Zach and Josh, always reach for them with both hands if I offer a platter of these yummy cookie bars when they come to visit.

1 full cup (3 ounces) dry quick-cooking oats
2 tablespoons Brown Sugar Twin
⅔ cup Carnation nonfat dry milk powder
1 teaspoon apple-pie spice
½ teaspoon baking soda
½ teaspoon baking powder
¼ cup raisins
1 cup unsweetened applesauce
1 tablespoon vanilla extract ☆
1 (8-ounce) package Philadelphia fat-free cream cheese
Sugar substitute to equal ¼ cup sugar
2 tablespoons (½ ounce) chopped pecans

Preheat oven to 350 degrees. In a large bowl, combine oats, Brown Sugar Twin, dry milk powder, apple-pie spice, baking soda, baking powder, and raisins. Add applesauce and 2 teaspoons vanilla extract. Mix well to combine. Pour batter into an 11-by-7-inch biscuit pan sprayed with butter-flavored cooking spray. Bake 20 to 25 minutes or until lightly browned. Cool 20 minutes in pan on wire rack. In a medium bowl, stir cream cheese with a spoon until soft. Add sugar substitute and remaining 1 teaspoon vanilla extract. Spread mixture over cooled oatmeal mixture. Sprinkle pecans evenly over top. Cut into 16 bars. Refrigerate leftovers.

Each serving equals:

HE: ½ Bread • ½ Fruit • ½ Protein • ½ Fat • ¼ Skim Milk • 8 Optional Calories

130 Calories • 2 gm Fat • 8 gm Protein • 20 gm Carbohydrate • 243 mg Sodium • 2 gm Fiber

DIABETIC: 1 Starch • ½ Fruit • ½ Meat

Orange Pudding Treats

Serves 4 ❄

If you loved the orange ice cream pushups of your youth, then you will definitely love this easy pudding. Cliff would be thrilled if I served this to him once a week—*forever.* But no such luck, as I'm always trying new recipes for my books and newsletter. Of course, he won't turn down an invitation from you if you promise him a dishful. . . .

1 (4-serving) package Jell-O sugar-free instant vanilla pudding mix
⅔ cup Carnation nonfat dry milk powder
1 cup unsweetened orange juice
¾ cup Yoplait plain fat-free yogurt
1 cup (one 11-ounce can) canned mandarin oranges, rinsed and drained
¼ cup Cool Whip Lite

In a medium bowl, combine dry pudding mix and dry milk powder. Add orange juice and yogurt. Mix well using a wire whisk. Blend in mandarin oranges. Spoon mixture into 4 dessert dishes. Top each with 1 tablespoon Cool Whip Lite. Refrigerate at least 15 minutes.

Each serving equals:

HE: 1 Fruit • ¾ Skim Milk • ¼ Slider • 12 Optional Calories

149 Calories • 1 gm Fat • 7 gm Protein • 28 gm Carbohydrate • 409 mg Sodium • 1 gm Fiber

DIABETIC: 1 Fruit • 1 Skim Milk

New England Pumpkin Raisin Pie

Serves 8 ❄

The addition of the raisins and maple syrup takes tried-and-true pumpkin pie to a new level of taste. Don't save this just for Thanksgiving—enjoy a piece of the Northeast all year round. Besides, no-bake pumpkin pies just don't get any easier!

1 (4-serving) package Jell-O sugar-free instant butterscotch pudding mix
⅔ cup Carnation nonfat dry milk powder
1 teaspoon pumpkin-pie spice
2 cups (one 16-ounce can) canned pumpkin
¼ cup Cary's sugar-free maple syrup
½ cup raisins
1 (6-ounce) Keebler graham-cracker piecrust
¾ cup Cool Whip Lite
2 tablespoons (½ ounce) chopped pecans

In a large bowl, combine dry pudding mix, dry milk powder, and pumpkin-pie spice. Add pumpkin and maple syrup. Mix well using a wire whisk. Stir in raisins. Pour mixture into piecrust. Evenly spread Cool Whip Lite over pumpkin mixture. Sprinkle pecans evenly over top. Refrigerate at least 2 hours. Cut into 8 pieces.

Each serving equals:

HE: ½ Bread • ½ Vegetable • ½ Fruit • ¼ Skim Milk • ¼ Fat • 1 Slider • 8 Optional Calories

219 Calories • 7 gm Fat • 4 gm Protein • 35 gm Carbohydrate • 309 mg Sodium • 3 gm Fiber

DIABETIC: 1½ Starch • 1 Fat • ½ Fruit

Raspberry Cream Treats

Serves 4 ❄

This easy dessert allows those "jewels of summer" to shine. When the farm stands are brimming with the ripest of the harvest, I could eat this every single day.

1 (4-serving) package Jell-O sugar-free instant vanilla pudding mix
2 cups skim milk
¾ cup fresh raspberries
½ teaspoon almond extract

In a medium bowl, combine dry pudding mix and skim milk. Mix well using a wire whisk. Blend in raspberries and almond extract. Evenly spoon mixture into 4 dessert dishes. Refrigerate at least 30 minutes.

Each serving equals:

HE: ½ Skim Milk • ¼ Fruit • 16 Optional Calories

76 Calories • 0 gm Fat • 4 gm Protein • 15 gm Carbohydrate • 255 mg Sodium • 0 gm Fiber

DIABETIC: ½ Skim Milk • ½ Fruit

S'Mores Pudding

Serves 4 ❄

A dish of this is *almost* like sitting around the campfire melting marshmallows for your graham cracker treats. Best of all, you don't even have to leave home. Yes, you may miss sitting under the stars, but remember, no mosquitoes either!

1 (4-serving) package Jell-O sugar-free instant butterscotch pudding mix
⅔ cup Carnation nonfat dry milk powder
1½ cups water
¼ cup (½ ounce) mini marshmallows
2 tablespoons (½ ounce) mini chocolate chips
6 (2½-inch) graham crackers, broken into pieces

In a large bowl, combine dry pudding mix and dry milk powder. Add water. Mix well with a wire whisk. Stir in marshmallows, chocolate chips, and graham cracker pieces. Evenly spoon pudding mixture into 4 dessert dishes. Refrigerate at least 30 minutes.

Each serving equals:

HE: ½ Skim Milk • ½ Bread • ½ Slider • 10 Optional Calories

138 Calories • 2 gm Fat • 5 gm Protein • 25 gm Carbohydrate • 427 mg Sodium • 0 gm Fiber

DIABETIC: 1½ Starch

Soda Fountain Delight

Serves 4

If this doesn't bring back memories of a childhood trip to the local drugstore for a tasty soda, I don't know what will. The combination of cherry, pineapple, and cola is so irresistible, I'm betting this will become a staple in your "goodies collection."

1 (4-serving) package Jell-O sugar-free cherry gelatin
1 cup (one 8-ounce can) canned crushed pineapple, packed in its own juice, undrained
1 cup Diet Coke
¾ cup Yoplait plain fat-free yogurt
¼ cup Cool Whip Lite
2 maraschino cherries, halved

Place dry gelatin in a medium bowl. In a small saucepan, heat crushed pineapple with juice to boiling. Pour over gelatin. Stir until gelatin is dissolved. Add Diet Coke and mix well until foam subsides. Refrigerate until mixture starts to thicken, about 30 minutes. Add yogurt and mix well using a wire whisk. Spoon mixture into 4 sundae dishes. Refrigerate at least 1 hour. Just before serving, top each with 1 tablespoon Cool Whip Lite and garnish with ½ maraschino cherry.

Each serving equals:
HE: ½ Fruit • ¼ Skim Milk • ¼ Slider • 2 Optional Calories

---

85 Calories • 1 gm Fat • 4 gm Protein • 15 gm Carbohydrate • 90 mg Sodium • 0 gm Fiber

---

DIABETIC: 1 Fruit

South Seas Chocolate Tarts

Serves 6 ❄

It just doesn't get any better than a chocolate and banana duo. Add a touch of coconut, and you have a real winner. I can feel those tropical breezes now. . . .

6 Keebler single-serve graham cracker shells
2 cups sliced bananas (2 medium)
1 (4-serving) package Jell-O sugar-free instant chocolate pudding mix
⅔ cup Carnation nonfat dry milk powder
1½ cups water
¼ teaspoon coconut extract
6 tablespoons Cool Whip Lite
2 teaspoons flaked coconut

Evenly divide sliced bananas among graham cracker shells. In a medium bowl, combine dry pudding mix and dry milk powder. Add water and coconut extract. Mix well using a wire whisk. Spoon mixture evenly over bananas. In a small bowl, combine Cool Whip Lite and flaked coconut. Evenly garnish each tart with Cool Whip Lite mixture. Refrigerate at least one hour.

Each serving equals:
HE: 1 Bread • ⅓ Fruit • ⅓ Skim Milk • ½ Slider • 11 Optional Calories

---

202 Calories • 6 gm Fat • 5 gm Protein • 32 gm Carbohydrate • 326 mg Sodium • 2 gm Fiber

---

DIABETIC: 1 Starch • 1 Fat • ½ Fruit

Wacky Spice Cake

Serves 8 ❄

Any cake that doesn't have sugar, oil, or eggs listed as ingredients can't be called anything *but* wacky. Try it—you may like it!

1½ cups flour
½ cup Sprinkle Sweet or *Sugar Twin*
¼ teaspoon salt
1 teaspoon baking soda
2 teaspoons pumpkin-pie spice
½ cup unsweetened applesauce
¾ cup water
1 tablespoon vinegar
2 teaspoons vanilla extract
6 tablespoons raisins

Preheat oven to 350 degrees. In a large bowl, combine flour, Sprinkle Sweet, salt, baking soda, and pumpkin-pie spice. In a small bowl, combine applesauce, water, vinegar, vanilla extract, and raisins. Add applesauce mixture to flour mixture. Mix gently to combine. Pour batter into an 8-by-8-inch cake pan sprayed with butter-flavored cooking spray. Bake 20 to 25 minutes or until cake tests done. Cool on wire rack.

Each serving equals:
HE: 1 Bread • ½ Fruit • 6 Optional Calories

120 Calories • 0 gm Fat • 3 gm Protein • 27 gm Carbohydrate • 164 mg Sodium • 1 gm Fiber

DIABETIC: 1 Starch • ½ Fruit

HINT: Good served with Cool Whip Lite. If using, don't forget to count the few additional calories.

Wonderful Butterscotch Treasure Pie

Serves 8

The butterscotch lovers in your life will put this *wonderful* pie on the top of their dessert list. The "crunchies" on the top are a feast for both their eyes and tastebuds.

2 (4-serving) packages Jell-O sugar-free instant butterscotch pudding mix
1⅓ cups Carnation nonfat dry milk powder
2½ cups water
1 teaspoon coconut extract ☆
1 (6-ounce) Keebler graham-cracker piecrust
¾ cup Cool Whip Lite
2 tablespoons flaked coconut
2 tablespoons (½ ounce) chopped pecans
1 tablespoon (¼ ounce) mini chocolate chips

In a medium bowl, combine dry pudding mixes and dry milk powder. Add water and ½ teaspoon coconut extract. Mix well using a wire whisk. Spread pudding mixture into piecrust. Refrigerate while preparing topping. In a small bowl, combine Cool Whip Lite and remaining ½ teaspoon coconut extract. Frost pie with topping mixture. Evenly sprinkle coconut, pecans, and chocolate chips over the top. Refrigerate at least 1 hour. Cut into 8 pieces.

Each serving equals:
HE: ½ Bread • ½ Skim Milk • ¼ Fat • 1 Slider

208 Calories • 8 gm Fat • 5 gm Protein • 29 gm Carbohydrate • 530 mg Sodium • 1 gm Fiber

DIABETIC: 2 Starch • 1 Fat

Note: This is a bonus recipe, not included in any of the week's menus. Isn't it *wonderful* to find an extra dessert recipe and have it be healthy at that?!

This and That

Apple Orchard Lemonade
Banana Nog
Blueberry "Ice Cream"
Breakfast Bread Pudding
Breakfast-in-Hand
Candy Drops
Carrot-Raisin Muffins
Cheese 'n' Fruit English
Cheesy Popcorn Snack
Chocolate Chip Drop Cookies
"Danish" Treat
Fruity-Cheese Sandwich
Grande Roma Dip
Ham-Spinach Dip
"Homemade" Limeade
Jo's Granola
Lemon Pancakes with Blueberry Sauce
Mexican Hot Chocolate
Mocha
Olé Scrambled Eggs
Orange Jo
Paradise Yogurt
Party Mix
Peach Melba Daiquiri
Peanut Butter and Jelly Pizza Snack
Potato Chips
Strawberry Shake
Stuffed Graham Crackers

Apple Orchard Lemonade

Serves 8 (1 cup)

I've always loved lemonade, and I'm a big fan of apple juice too. But until I "made-over" a recipe for a reader's favorite summer thirst quencher, I hadn't imagined enjoying the two tastes together! I'm sure you'll find this blend wonderfully refreshing—and a real treat to enjoy all year long.

2 cups unsweetened apple juice
6 cups cold water
1 tub Crystal Light Lemonade mix

In a large pitcher, combine apple juice and water. Add dry lemonade mix. Stir well to dissolve. Pour over ice into tall glasses.

Each serving equals:
HE: ½ Fruit

28 Calories • 0 gm Fat • 0 gm Protein • 7 gm Carbohydrate • 2 mg Sodium • 0 gm Fiber

DIABETIC: ½ Fruit

Banana Nog

Serves 4 (1 cup)

This is both a healthy and refreshing way to chase your thirst away. I think you will be pleased by the unusual flavor combinations in this nog. So good—and so good for you!

1½ cups Yoplait plain fat-free yogurt
1 cup Ocean Spray reduced-calorie cranapple juice
1 cup sliced banana (1 medium)
½ teaspoon almond extract
Sugar substitute to equal 2 tablespoons sugar
2-3 ice cubes

In a blender container, combine yogurt, cranapple juice, sliced banana, almond extract, and sugar substitute. Cover and process on BLEND until smooth. Add ice cubes, one at a time, blending until smooth. Pour into 4 glasses.

Each serving equals:
HE: ¾ Fruit • ½ Skim Milk • 3 Optional Calories

88 Calories • 0 gm Fat • 5 gm Protein • 17 gm Carbohydrate • 67 mg Sodium • 1 gm Fiber

DIABETIC: 1 Fruit

Blueberry "Ice Cream"

Serves 1 ❄

Okay, this isn't Ben & Jerry's, but it sure hits the spot when an ice cream craving appears from out of nowhere! Get creative and start "blending" the flavor of the week in your own kitchen.

⅓ cup Carnation nonfat dry milk powder
Sugar substitute to equal ¼ cup sugar
⅔ cup water
1 teaspoon almond extract
1 cup frozen unsweetened blueberries

In blender container, combine dry milk powder, sugar substitute, water, and almond extract. Process on HIGH 10 seconds. Add frozen blueberries. Process on HIGH 15 to 20 seconds or until thick.

Each serving equals:

HE: 1⅓ Fruit • 1 Skim Milk • 12 Optional Calories

173 Calories • 1 gm Fat • 7 gm Protein • 34 gm Carbohydrate • 201 mg Sodium • 1 gm Fiber

DIABETIC: 1½ Fruit • 1 Skim Milk

Breakfast Bread Pudding

Serves 4

Bread pudding is my all-time most favorite dessert. I just took it one step further and came up with a way to enjoy it early in the morning, while still being sure to include all the essentials of a well-balanced breakfast.

4 slices toasted reduced-calorie bread
2 tablespoons Peter Pan reduced-fat peanut butter
2 tablespoons spreadable fruit spread (any flavor)
1 (4-serving) package Jell-O sugar-free instant vanilla pudding mix
2 cups skim milk

Spread each slice of toast with 1½ teaspoons of both peanut butter and spreadable fruit spread. Cut into small cubes. Evenly divide cubes in 4 dessert dishes. In a medium bowl, combine dry pudding mix and skim milk. Mix well using a wire whisk. Pour ½ cup pudding mixture over toast cubes in each dish. Cover and refrigerate at least 1 hour.

Each serving equals:

HE: ½ Protein • ½ Bread • ½ Fat • ½ Fruit • ½ Skim Milk • ¼ Slider • 5 Optional Calories

180 Calories • 4 gm Fat • 9 gm Protein • 27 gm Carbohydrate • 437 mg Sodium • 1 gm Fiber

DIABETIC: 1½ Starch • 1 Meat • ½ Skim Milk

HINT: Best if made the night before.

Breakfast-in-Hand

Serves 1

Even if you only have sixty seconds before you've got to dash out the door, you have enough time to fix this easy breakfast. Then you can eat it on the run as you head for work or school.

2 slices reduced-calorie bread
1 tablespoon apple butter
1 tablespoon Peter Pan reduced-fat peanut butter
½ cup sliced banana (½ medium)

Spread apple butter on one slice bread. Spread peanut butter on other slice. Place banana slices on peanut butter. Cover with apple butter slice. Eat at once or cover and refrigerate until ready to serve.

Each serving equals:

HE: 1 Bread • 1 Protein • 1 Fat • 1 Fruit • 15 Optional Calories

268 Calories • 8 gm Fat • 10 gm Protein • 39 gm Carbohydrate • 242 mg Sodium • 3 gm Fiber

DIABETIC: 1 Starch • 1 Meat • 1 Fat • 1 Fruit

HINT: I purchase the smallest banana I can (sometimes called a finger banana). I use the entire banana and count as 1½ Fruit.

Candy Drops

Serves 6 (4 each) ❄

Let the kids (of all ages) help you make these quick yet tasty treats. They are the closest thing to the "real thing" without going to the candy store.

¼ cup Peter Pan reduced-fat peanut butter
⅔ cup Carnation nonfat dry milk powder
1 tablespoon unsweetened cocoa
2 tablespoons Sprinkle Sweet or *Sugar Twin*
⅓ cup water
1½ cups (2¼ ounces) crushed corn flakes
¼ cup raisins

In a medium bowl, combine peanut butter, dry milk powder, cocoa, Sprinkle Sweet, and water. Stir in corn flakes and raisins. Place waxed paper on cookie sheet. Drop mixture by teaspoonfuls to form 24 drops. Refrigerate 30 minutes. Cover and refrigerate leftovers.

Each serving equals:

HE: ⅔ Protein • ⅔ Fat • ½ Bread • ⅓ Fruit • ⅓ Skim Milk • 5 Optional Calories

157 Calories • 5 gm Fat • 6 gm Protein • 22 gm Carbohydrate • 196 mg Sodium • 2 gm Fiber

DIABETIC: 1 Starch • ½ Meat • ½ Fat • ½ Fruit

Carrot-Raisin Muffins

Serves 8 ❄

These wonderful muffins were conceived when a subscriber asked me to make over her husband's favorite breakfast treat. I shared my Healthy Exchanges version in the newsletter. Then, a few months later, I received a letter from another subscriber telling me her granddaughter had stirred up a batch and entered them in the county fair—and won a blue ribbon!

1½ cups flour
1 (4-serving) package Jell-O sugar-free instant vanilla pudding mix
¼ cup Sprinkle Sweet or *Sugar Twin*
1 teaspoon baking powder
1 teaspoon baking soda
1 teaspoon pumpkin-pie spice
1 cup grated carrots
½ cup raisins
½ cup unsweetened applesauce
2 tablespoons + 2 teaspoons vegetable oil
1 teaspoon vanilla extract
2 eggs or *equivalent in egg substitute*
¼ cup skim milk

Preheat oven to 350 degrees. In a large bowl, combine flour, dry pudding mix, Sprinkle Sweet, baking powder, baking soda, and pumpkin-pie spice. Add carrots and raisins. Mix well. In a small bowl, combine applesauce, vegetable oil, vanilla extract, eggs, and skim milk. Add to flour mixture. Mix just until combined. Spray muffin tins with butter-flavored cooking spray or line with muffin liners. Fill 8 muffin wells. Bake 20 to 22 minutes or until muffins test done. Cool in pan 5 minutes. Remove from pan and continue cooling on wire racks.

Each serving equals:

HE: 1 Bread • 1 Fat • ⅔ Fruit • ¼ Protein (limited) • 15 Optional Calories

---

210 Calories • 6 gm Fat • 5 gm Protein • 34 gm Carbohydrate • 304 mg Sodium • 2 gm Fiber

---

DIABETIC: 1 Starch • 1 Fruit • 1 Fat

HINT: Fill unused muffin wells with water. It protects the muffin tin and ensures even baking.

Cheese 'n' Fruit English

Serves 1

Talk about easy—this one has to win the prize! Stirring the fruit spread into the fat-free cream cheese makes a special topping for any breakfast bread.

2 tablespoons Philadelphia fat-free cream cheese
1 tablespoon spreadable fruit spread (any flavor)
1 English muffin, split

In a small saucer, combine cream cheese and spreadable fruit spread. Toast English muffin halves. Evenly spread cream cheese mixture over toasted halves. Serve at once.

Each serving equals:

HE: 2 Bread • 1 Fruit • ½ Protein

217 Calories • 1 gm Fat • 12 gm Protein • 40 gm Carbohydrate • 479 mg Sodium • 2 gm Fiber

DIABETIC: 2 Starch • ½ Fruit • ½ Meat

Cheesy Popcorn Snack

Serves 4 (1½ cups)

If you thought popcorn and cheese were both off the "good-for-you" list forever, then dig into this flavorful snack . . . without any guilt.

¼ cup grated Kraft American cheese (¾ ounce)
1 tablespoon + 1 teaspoon melted reduced-calorie margarine
1 teaspoon chili seasoning mix
1 teaspoon dried parsley flakes
6 cups air-popped popcorn
I Can't Believe It's Not Butter Air Pump Spray

In a small bowl, combine American cheese, margarine, chili seasoning mix, and parsley flakes. In a large bowl, quickly spray popcorn with butter-flavored spray. Add cheese mixture. Toss gently to coat popcorn. Store in airtight container.

Each serving equals:

HE: ½ Bread • ½ Fat • ¼ Protein

75 Calories • 3 gm Fat • 3 gm Protein • 9 gm Carbohydrate • 93 mg Sodium • 1 gm Fiber

DIABETIC: ½ Starch • ½ Fat

Chocolate Chip Drop Cookies

Serves 12 (3 each) ❄

Mrs. Fields' they're not, but for a cookie without sugar or tons of butter, these are quite good. Notice that I've planned it so a realistic serving is *three* cookies. Doesn't it just get you when you see recipes that *assume* anyone would be satisfied with only one?

⅓ cup + 1 tablespoon reduced-calorie margarine
2 tablespoons unsweetened applesauce
1 egg or *equivalent in egg substitute*
1 teaspoon vanilla extract
½ cup Sprinkle Sweet or *Sugar Twin*
2 tablespoons Brown Sugar Twin
1 cup + 2 tablespoons flour
½ teaspoon baking soda
¼ teaspoon salt
⅓ cup (1½ ounces) mini chocolate chips
½ cup (2 ounces) chopped walnuts

Preheat oven to 375 degrees. In a medium bowl, combine margarine, applesauce, and egg. Mix well using a wire whisk until blended. Blend in vanilla extract, Sprinkle Sweet, and Brown Sugar Twin. Add flour, baking soda, and salt. Mix well to combine using a large spoon. Stir in chocolate chips and walnuts. Drop by teaspoonfuls to form 36 cookies on cookie sheets sprayed with butter-flavored cooking spray. Bake 9 to 11 minutes. Don't overbake! Cool on wire rack.

Each serving equals:

HE: 1 Fat • ½ Bread • ¼ Protein • ¼ Slider • 10 Optional Calories

---

131 Calories • 7 gm Fat • 3 gm Protein • 14 gm Carbohydrate • 104 mg Sodium • 1 gm Fiber

---

DIABETIC: 1 Starch • 1 Fat

"Danish" Treat

Serves 1

Don't just think of this tasty treat only for breakfast. It's a great choice for a mid-afternoon snack.

1 slice reduced-calorie bread
1½ teaspoons Philadelphia fat-free cream cheese
¼ teaspoon cinnamon
1½ tablespoons raisins

Toast bread. Spread cream cheese evenly over bread. Evenly sprinkle cinnamon and raisins over top. Serve at once.

Each serving equals:

HE: ¾ Fruit • ½ Bread • ¼ Protein

---

140 Calories • 0 gm Fat • 8 gm Protein • 27 gm Carbohydrate • 253 mg Sodium • 1 gm Fiber

---

DIABETIC: 1 Fruit • ½ Starch

Fruity-Cheese Sandwich

Serves 1

This is my usual "snack of choice" when I get the hungries about 4:30 P.M. It's just enough to fill my tummy without going into overload.

- *2 slices reduced-calorie bread*
- *1 tablespoon spreadable fruit spread (any flavor)*
- *1½ teaspoons Philadelphia fat-free cream cheese*

Spread fruit spread on one slice of bread and cream cheese on the other. Make into a sandwich. Serve at once or cover and refrigerate until ready to serve.

Each serving equals:

HE: 1 Bread • 1 Fruit • ¼ Protein

140 Calories • 0 gm Fat • 8 gm Protein • 27 gm Carbohydrate • 274 mg Sodium • 2 gm Fiber

DIABETIC: 1 Starch • 1 Fruit

Grande Roma Dip

Serves 8 (full ¼ cup)

My son James loves the combination of Mexican and Italian flavors in this easy dip. By adding the Italian seasoning to the Mexican salsa you really have the best of two worlds! P.S.: This is another dip that's just as good on a baked potato as it is used in the conventional way.

- *¾ cup Yoplait plain fat-free yogurt*
- *⅓ cup Carnation nonfat dry milk powder*
- *¼ cup Kraft fat-free mayonnaise*
- *1 cup chunky salsa*
- *1 teaspoon Italian seasoning*

In a medium bowl, combine yogurt, dry milk powder, and mayonnaise. Stir in salsa and Italian seasoning. Mix well to combine. Cover and refrigerate at least 30 minutes.

Each serving equals:

HE: ¼ Skim Milk • ¼ Vegetable • 10 Optional Calories

28 calories • 0 gm Fat • 2 gm Protein • 5 gm Carbohydrate • 194 mg Sodium • 0 gm Fiber

DIABETIC: 1 Vegetable

Ham-Spinach Dip

Serves 6 (½ cup)

My daughter, Becky, went wild over this scrumptious dip. I based it on her favorite dip and added a few of my own special touches. If you have any left over, it's great on a hot baked potato.

1 (8-ounce) package Philadelphia fat-free cream cheese
¾ cup Yoplait plain fat-free yogurt
⅓ cup Carnation nonfat dry milk powder
½ cup Kraft fat-free mayonnaise
1 teaspoon Italian seasoning
1 full cup (6 ounces) finely diced Dubuque 97% fat-free or *any extra-lean ham*
1 (10-ounce) package frozen chopped spinach, thawed and thoroughly *drained*

In a medium bowl, stir cream cheese with a spoon until soft. Add yogurt, dry milk powder, mayonnaise, and Italian seasoning. Continue mixing until well blended. Add diced ham and drained spinach. Mix gently to combine. Cover and refrigerate at least 30 minutes.

Each serving equals:

HE: 1⅓ Protein • ½ Vegetable • ⅓ Skim Milk • 14 Optional Calories

---

109 Calories • 1 gm Fat • 13 gm Protein • 12 gm Carbohydrate • 452 mg Sodium • 1 gm Fiber

---

DIABETIC: 1½ Meat • 2 Vegetable

"Homemade" Limeade

Serves 8 (1 cup)

This gets my vote for the most satisfying thirst quencher you can stir up in a pitcher. Even if it's 100 degrees in the shade, a glass of this will put a smile on everyone's face.

1 tub Crystal Light sugar-free limeade mix
8 cups water
¼ of a lemon cut into chunks, including skin and seeds

In a large pitcher, combine dry limeade mix and water. Mix well using a long spoon. Pour 2 cups of prepared limeade into blender; add lemon chunks and blend on HIGH for 30 to 45 seconds. Pour back into the pitcher of limeade mixture and mix well. Serve over ice and enjoy!

Each serving equals:

HE: 1 Optional Calorie

---

1 Calorie • 0 gm Fat • 0 gm Protein • 0 gm Carbohydrate • less than 1 mg Sodium • 0 gm Fiber

---

DIABETIC: Free food

Jo's Granola

Serves 1

This is my favorite way to eat cereal. By adding my extra crunches to plain old corn flakes, I end up with something that's anything but plain! It's the perfect wake-up call for your taste buds.

- *¾ cup (¾ ounce) corn flakes*
- *1 tablespoon raisins*
- *½ cup sliced banana (½ medium)*
- *2 teaspoons chopped pecans*
- *2 tablespoons Brown Sugar Twin*
- *1 cup skim milk*

In a cereal bowl, combine corn flakes, raisins, sliced banana, pecans, and Brown Sugar Twin. Add skim milk. Munch away.

Each serving equals:

HE: 1½ Fruit • 1 Bread • 1 Skim Milk • ⅔ Fat • 9 Optional Calories

292 Calories • 4 gm Fat • 11 gm Protein • 53 gm Carbohydrate • 289 mg Sodium • 3 gm Fiber

DIABETIC: 1½ Fruit • 1 Starch • 1 Skim Milk • ½ Fat

HINT: I purchase the smallest banana I can (sometimes called a finger banana) and use the entire banana with my cereal. I would then count my Fruit as 2. Unless you split your medium banana with someone, what are you going to do with the leftover?

Lemon Pancakes with Blueberry Sauce

Serves 8 ❄

My grandson Zach's all-time favorite breakfast treat. He's crazy about both pancakes and blueberries. I whipped up these when he was spending the weekend with Grandma and Grandpa. It was pure pleasure to see that perfect child's face all smeared with blueberry sauce as he gobbled his hotcakes down.

- *2 (4-serving) packages Jell-O sugar-free lemon gelatin* ☆
- *1 (4-serving) package Jell-O sugar-free vanilla cook-and-serve pudding mix*
- *2 cups water* ☆
- *1½ cups fresh* or *frozen blueberries, thawed and well drained*
- *1½ cups Bisquick reduced-fat baking mix*
- *⅓ cup Carnation nonfat dry milk powder*
- *2 eggs* or *equivalent in egg substitute*
- *¾ cup Yoplait plain fat-free yogurt*

In a medium saucepan, combine 1 package dry gelatin, dry pudding mix, and 1½ cups water. Add blueberries. Cook over medium heat, stirring often until mixture thickens and comes to a boil. Remove from heat.

In a medium bowl, combine baking mix, remaining 1 package dry gelatin, and dry milk powder.

In a small bowl, slightly beat eggs. Add yogurt and remaining ½ cup water. Mix well to combine. Add egg mixture to baking mix mixture. Stir gently just to combine. Spray a large skillet with butter-flavored cooking spray. For each pancake, pour a full ¼ cup batter onto skillet. Cook until lightly brown on bottom (1 to 2 minutes). Turn pancakes; continue cooking until browned on both sides. Keep browned pancakes warm while preparing remaining pancakes.

When serving, spoon a full ¼ cup warm blueberry sauce over each pancake.

Each serving equals:

HE: 1 Bread • ¼ Skim Milk • ¼ Protein (limited) • ¼ Fruit • 18 Optional Calories

155 Calories • 3 gm Fat • 7 gm Protein • 25 gm Carbohydrate • 365 mg Sodium • 2 gm Fiber

DIABETIC: 1 Starch • ½ Fruit • 1 Meat

Mexican Hot Chocolate

Serves 2

Take a sip of this full-bodied chocolate nectar, and you just may feel ready for a fiesta.

- *⅔ cup Carnation nonfat dry milk powder*
- *¼ cup Sprinkle Sweet* or *Sugar Twin*
- *¼ cup Nestlé's Quik sugar-free instant chocolate drink mix*
- *2 cups boiling water*
- *½ teaspoon cinnamon*
- *1 teaspoon vanilla extract*

In 4-cup glass measure, combine dry milk powder, Sprinkle Sweet, and Nestlé's Quik. Add boiling water. Mix well to combine. Stir in cinnamon and vanilla extract. Mix well with wire whisk until foamy. Pour into 2 large mugs.

Each serving equals:

HE: 1 Skim Milk

73 Calories • 1 gm Fat • 5 gm Protein • 11 gm Carbohydrate • 153 mg Sodium • 0 gm Fiber

DIABETIC: 1 Skim Milk

Mocha

Serves 1

My daughter, Becky, suggested this easy way to stir up a cup of flavored coffee. I don't care for the taste of coffee myself, but I found this quite tasty.

⅓ cup Carnation nonfat dry milk powder
2 tablespoons Sprinkle Sweet or *Sugar Twin*
2 tablespoons Nestlé's Quik sugar-free instant chocolate drink mix
1 (8 ounce) cup hot coffee
1 tablespoon Cool Whip Lite

In a large mug, combine dry milk powder, Sprinkle Sweet, and Nestlé's Quik. Add hot coffee. Mix well to combine. Top with 1 tablespoon Cool Whip Lite and enjoy.

Each serving equals:
HE: 1 Skim Milk • 8 Optional Calories

81 Calories • 1 gm Fat • 6 gm Protein • 12 gm Carbohydrate • 161 mg Sodium • 0 gm Fiber

DIABETIC: 1 Skim Milk

Olé Scrambled Eggs

Serves 4

Cliff said he'd get up early any day of the week for this delectable egg dish. Since I usually get up between 3:30 and 4:00 A.M., he *does* mean early!

4 eggs or *equivalent in egg substitute*
2 tablespoons skim milk
½ teaspoon lemon pepper
½ cup chunky salsa
3 tablespoons (¾ ounce) shredded Kraft reduced-fat Cheddar cheese
¼ cup Land O Lakes fat-free sour cream

In a medium bowl, combine eggs, skim milk, and lemon pepper. Stir with fork until fluffy. Pour mixture into a large skillet sprayed with butter-flavored cooking spray. Cook over medium heat, stirring as needed, until cooked through. For each serving, spoon ¼ of egg mixture onto plate. Top each with 2 tablespoons salsa, full 2 teaspoons Cheddar cheese, and 1 tablespoon sour cream.

Each serving equals:
HE: 1¼ Protein (limited) • ¼ Vegetable • 15 Optional Calories

106 Calories • 6 gm Fat • 9 gm Protein • 4 gm Carbohydrate • 144 mg Sodium • 0 gm Fiber

DIABETIC: 1 Meat • 1 Vegetable

Orange Jo

Serves 4

Whip this up after a hard day's work, and you'll feel like a million bucks. If this creamy potion doesn't "make it all better," I don't know what will.

2 cups unsweetened orange juice
1½ cups Diet 7UP
1 (4-serving) package Jell-O sugar-free vanilla cook-and-serve pudding mix
¼ cup Cool Whip Lite
½ cup crushed ice

In blender container, combine orange juice, Diet 7UP, and dry pudding mix. Process on BLEND 15 seconds. Add Cool Whip Lite and process on BLEND another 15 seconds. Add ice gradually and process on HIGH until blended. Pour into 4 glasses.

Each serving equals:
HE: 1 Fruit • ¼ Slider • 8 Optional Calories

85 Calories • 1 gm Fat • 1 gm Protein • 18 gm Carbohydrate • 148 mg Sodium • 1 gm Fiber

DIABETIC: 1 Fruit

Paradise Yogurt

Serves 4 (¾ cup)

If you keep this almost effortless yogurt goody on hand in the fridge all the time, you will have the perfect foil the next time hunger strikes. A dish of this is almost like paradise on earth.

3 cups Yoplait plain fat-free yogurt
1 tub Crystal Light tropical punch beverage mix

In a large bowl, combine yogurt and dry beverage mix. Mix well. Store in a covered container in refrigerator.

Each serving equals:
HE: 1 Skim Milk

92 Calories • 0 gm Fat • 10 gm Protein • 13 gm Carbohydrate • 115 mg Sodium • 0 gm Fiber

DIABETIC: 1 Skim Milk

HINT: You can also use Lemon Crystal Light for lemon-flavored yogurt or make any other flavor you choose.

Party Mix

Serves 16 (1 full cup) ❄

A crunchy bowl of cereal mix has always been on Cliff's "most preferred" list of snacks. I stirred this up for him after he began complaining that I was always making up special recipes for others, but none just for him. He sure quieted down after his first munch of this combo. Notice what I replaced half the margarine with—isn't it great what we can do with that fat-free dressing besides just pouring it on our lettuce salads?

½ cup reduced-calorie margarine
½ cup Kraft fat-free Italian dressing
2 tablespoons Worcestershire sauce
½ teaspoon garlic powder
5 cups (4½ ounces) Rice Chex
5 cups (7½ ounces) Wheat Chex
5 cups (4 ounces) Cheerios
2½ cups (5 ounces) Keebler reduced-sodium and fat-free pretzels, coarsely broken

Preheat oven to 250 degrees. In a medium saucepan, combine margarine, Italian dressing, Worcestershire sauce, and garlic powder. Cook over medium heat, stirring constantly, 3 minutes. In a very large bowl, combine Rice Chex, Wheat Chex, Cheerios, and pretzels. Drizzle slightly cooled margarine mixture over top. Mix well. Spray 2 large cookie sheets or jelly-roll pans with butter-flavored cooking spray. Evenly spread mixture in pans. Bake 60 minutes, stirring every 15 minutes. Store in airtight container.

Each serving equals:

HE: 1¾ Bread • ¾ Fat • 2 Optional Calories

163 Calories • 3 gm Fat • 3 gm Protein • 31 gm Carbohydrate • 373 mg Sodium • 2 gm Fiber

DIABETIC: 2 Starch

Peach Melba Daiquiri

Serves 4 (1 cup)

The combination of frozen peaches and sugar-free raspberry gelatin in this luscious drink is out of this world. The Diet Dew and rum extract replace the usual alcohol, so you don't even need a designated driver after enjoying a glass with friends.

2 cups Diet Mountain Dew
½ teaspoon rum extract
1 (4-serving) package Jell-O sugar-free raspberry gelatin
2 cups frozen unsweetened peach slices
½ cup ice cubes

In blender container, combine Diet Mountain Dew, rum extract, and dry gelatin. Process on HIGH 15 seconds. Add frozen peach slices and ice cubes. Continue processing on HIGH until mixture is smooth, about 30 to 45 seconds. Pour mixture into 4 glasses.

Each serving equals:

HE: 1 Fruit • 10 Optional Calories

48 Calories • 0 gm Fat • 2 gm Protein • 10 gm Carbohydrate • 72 mg Sodium • 1 gm Fiber

DIABETIC: 1 Fruit

Peanut Butter and Jelly Pizza Snack

Serves 1

I'm proud to admit I'm a full card-carrying member of the "I Love Peanut Butter" Club. While peanut butter may be high in protein, it's still high in fat, too, even the reduced-fat versions. I choose my times and places very selectively so that I can savor every precious bite. If the club took a vote, I bet this easy snack would be chosen #1!

1 slice reduced-calorie bread
1½ teaspoons Philadelphia fat-free cream cheese
¾ teaspoon Peter Pan reduced-fat peanut butter
1 teaspoon grape spreadable fruit spread

Toast bread slice. While warm, spread cream cheese over toast. Spread peanut butter evenly over cream cheese. Evenly spread grape spreadable fruit over top. Serve at once.

Each serving equals:

HE: ¾ Fat • ½ Bread • ⅓ Fruit • ¼ Protein

---

90 Calories • 2 gm Fat • 6 gm Protein • 12 gm Carbohydrate • 179 mg Sodium • 1 gm Fiber

---

DIABETIC: 1 Starch • ½ Fat

Potato Chips

Serves 4

My potato chip lovers truly love snacking on these easy potato chips—and they take just minutes to make up fresh. I bet your chip fans will too.

2 cups (10 ounces) raw, unpeeled potatoes
¼ teaspoon salt

Cut potatoes into very thin slices. Arrange slices in circle on microwave bacon-cooking rack sprayed with butter-flavored cooking spray. Sprinkle with salt. Cook on HIGH 5½ to 6½ minutes or until brown. Turn halfway through cooking time. Let stand 1 minute.

Each serving equals:

HE: ½ Bread

---

56 Calories • 0 gm Fat • 2 gm Protein • 12 gm Carbohydrate • 136 mg Sodium • 1 gm Fiber

---

DIABETIC: 1 Starch

HINTS: 1. If using Cuisinart blade, use #1.
2. If using a conventional oven, place potato slices on a cookie sheet sprayed with butter-flavored cooking spray, and bake at 400 degrees for about 20 minutes.

Strawberry Shake

Serves 1

This easy shake goes together almost as fast as you can say, "I'm hungry. What's to eat or drink around here?" Enjoy!

⅓ cup Carnation nonfat dry milk powder
Sugar substitute to equal 3 tablespoons sugar
1 cup water
½ teaspoon almond extract
¾ cup frozen unsweetened strawberries

In blender container, combine dry milk powder, sugar substitute, water, and almond extract. Process on HIGH 5 seconds. Add frozen strawberries. Process on HIGH until mixture is smooth and thick, about 30 seconds.

Each serving equals:

HE: 1 Skim Milk • ¾ Fruit

133 Calories • 1 gm Fat • 7 gm Protein • 24 gm Carbohydrate • 203 mg Sodium • 2 gm Fiber

DIABETIC: 1 Skim Milk • 1 Fruit

Stuffed Graham Crackers

Serves 4 ❄

Just the thought of peanut butter brings a smile to my mouth. I'd give this recipe 12 peanuts any day on a 10-peanut pleasure scale!

3 tablespoons Peter Pan reduced-fat peanut butter
2 tablespoons raisins
1 tablespoon flaked coconut
1 tablespoon quick rolled oats
8 (2½-inch) graham cracker squares

In a small bowl, combine peanut butter, raisins, coconut, and rolled oats. Mix well. Drop a tablespoonful of mixture onto 4 graham crackers. Top each with another graham cracker. Eat at once or store individually in Ziploc sandwich bags.

Each serving equals:

HE: ¾ Protein • ¾ Fat • ⅔ Bread • ¼ Fruit • 14 Optional Calories

157 Calories • 5 gm Fat • 5 gm Protein • 23 gm Carbohydrate • 164 mg Sodium • 1 gm Fiber

DIABETIC: 1½ Starch • 1 Meat • ½ Fat

Note: This is a bonus recipe, not included in any of the week's menus. I just had to make the last recipe in my book a bonus recipe, or "one for the road," as you travel to good health with me.

Index

I want to hear from you. . . .

Besides my family, the love of my life is creating "common folk" healthy recipes and solving everyday cooking questions in *The Healthy Exchanges Way.* Everyone who uses my recipes is considered part of the Healthy Exchanges Family, so please write to me if you have any questions, comments, or suggestions. I will do my best to answer. With your support, I'll continue to stir up even more recipes and cooking tips for the Family in the years to come.

Write to: JoAnna M. Lund
c/o Healthy Exchanges, Inc.
P.O. Box 124
DeWitt, IA 52742

If you prefer, you can fax me at 319-659-2126 or E-mail me at Healthyjo@aol.com.

JoAnna

Now That You've Seen *HELP: The Healthy Exchanges Lifetime Plan,* Why Not Order *The Healthy Exchanges Food Newsletter?*

If you enjoyed the recipes in this cookbook and would like to cook up even more of these "common folk" healthy dishes, you may want to subscribe to *The Healthy Exchanges Food Newsletter.*

This monthly 12-page newsletter contains 30-plus new recipes *every month* in such columns as:

- Reader Exchange
- Special Requests
- Recipe Makeover
- Micro Corner
- Dinner for Two
- Crock-Pot Luck
- Meatless Main Dishes
- Rise & Shine
- Brown Bagging It
- Snack Attack
- Side Dishes
- Main Dishes
- Desserts

In addition to all the recipes, other regular features include:

- The Editor's Motivational Corner
- Dining Out Question & Answer
- Cooking Question & Answer
- New Product Alert
- Success Profiles of Winners in the Losing Game

Just as in this cookbook, all *Healthy Exchanges Food Newsletter* recipes are calculated in three distinct ways: 1) Weight Loss Choices, 2) Calories with Fat and Fiber Grams, and 3) Diabetic Exchanges.

The cost for a one-year (12-issue) subscription (including a special Healthy Exchanges three-ring binder to store the newsletters) is $26.50. To order, simply complete the form and mail to us *or* call our toll-free number and pay with your VISA or MasterCard. (Please photocopy this order blank if you don't want to remove the page from the book.)

_____ Yes, I want to subscribe to *The Healthy Exchanges Food Newsletter*
$26.50 Yearly Subscription Cost . . . . $ _____

_____ Foreign orders please add $6.00 for money exchange and extra postage. . . . . $ _____

_____ I'm not sure, so please send me a sample copy at $2.50 . . . . $ _____

Total . . . . $ _____

Please make check payable to HEALTHY EXCHANGES or pay by VISA/MasterCard

CARD NUMBER: _____________________ EXPIRATION DATE: _____________

SIGNATURE: ____

Signature required for all credit card orders.

Or Order Toll-Free, using your credit card, at 1-800-766-8961

NAME: ____

ADDRESS: ____

CITY ______________ STATE _____ ZIP _____

TELEPHONE: (   ) ___________

If additional orders for the newsletter are to be sent to an address other than the one listed above, please use a separate sheet and attach to this form.

MAIL TO: HEALTHY EXCHANGES
P.O. BOX 124
DeWitt, IA 52742-0124

1-800-766-8961 For Customer Orders
1-319-659-8234 For Customer Service

Thank you for your order, and for choosing to become a part of the Healthy Exchanges family!